The Canadian Patient Safety Institute is pleased to endorse *Take as Directed*. This is a valuable tool to help Canadians navigate the health-care system safely.

— Hugh MacLeod, CEO
Canadian Patient Safety Institute

The authors provide helpful information that can guide Canadians on how to manage their health care, including safe medication use. ISMP Canada supports efforts that improve medication safety.

— Sylvia Hyland, RPh, BScPhm, MHSc
Vice President and Chief Operating Officer
Institute for Safe Medication Practices Canada

More Praise for *Take as Directed*

An excellent, in depth, yet thoroughly understandable read! Definitely targeted at the issue of medication error, but applicable to all who have occasion to enter the health-care system. I see this as an indispensible guide for all health-care sector navigators and providers. It provides easy-to-read, practical advice and is certainly one book I will have available for my patients.

— Ken Buchholz, Senior Physician Advisor
Nova Scotia Department of Health

Patients who want to get the best out of Canada's health-care system will benefit from reading *Take as Directed*. Church and MacKinnon, a family doctor and a pharmacist, have put together advice that will help every Canadian meet the challenges of working with doctors and pharmacists to use medications appropriately. The style of writing makes difficult topics easy to follow. Helping consumers to better understand and improve their use of health care is critical to maintaining a viable system.

— Jeff Poston, PhD, MRPharmS, Executive Director
Canadian Pharmacists Association

In *Take as Directed*, Church and MacKinnon have demystified for the patient the three primary centers where the delivery of health-care services takes place: the doctor's office, the pharmacy, and the hospital. Their "what's that behind the curtain" tour of these professional environments helps the patient see where mistakes can happen and how to better manage and ensure their own access to quality heath care. The authors' nine tips for navigating the health-care system in Canada apply equally to all patients around the world who must chase the tails of their professionals and be the squeaky wheel to ensure that proper treatment and follow up occurs. Church and MacKinnon have done a super job providing a practical guide for patients, particularly in the area of medication safety.

— Cathy Horton, Founder
FLAAME (Families Launching Action Against Medication Error)

TAKE AS DIRECTED

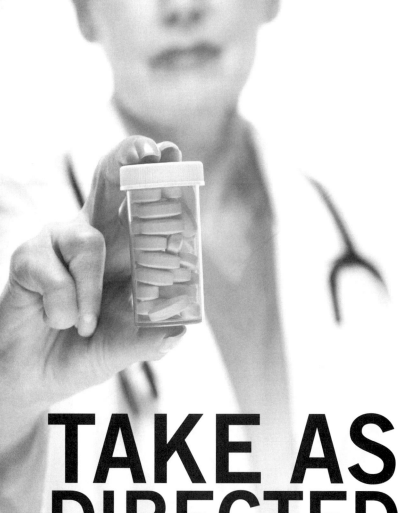

TAKE AS
DIRECTED

Your Prescription for
Safe Health Care in Canada

Rhonda Church, M.D. & Neil MacKinnon, Ph.D.

ECW Press

Published by ECW Press, 2120 Queen Street East, Suite 200,
Toronto, Ontario, Canada M4E 1E2
416.694.3348 / info@ecwpress.com

LIBRARY AND ARCHIVES CANADA CATALOGUING IN PUBLICATION

MacKinnon, Neil J. (Neil John), 1971-
Take as directed : your prescription for safe health care in
Canada / Neil MacKinnon and Rhonda Church.

Includes bibliographical references and index.
ISBN 978-1-55022-952-3

1. Drugs—Canada—Safety measures. 2. Pharmaceutical
services—Canada. 3. Patient education—Canada. I. Church,
Rhonda II. Title.

RM300.M33 2010   615'.10971   C2010-901370-0

Editor: Alison DeLory
Cover and text design: Tania Craan
Cover images: iStock photo
Typesetting: Mary Bowness
Printing: Webcom 1 2 3 4 5

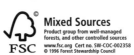

Mixed Sources
Product group from well-managed
forests, and other controlled sources
www.fsc.org Cert no. SW-COC-002358
© 1996 Forest Stewardship Council

The publication of *Take as Directed* has been generously supported by the Government of Ontario through Ontario Book Publishing Tax Credit, by the OMDC Book Fund, an initiative of the Ontario Media Development Corporation, and by the Government of Canada through the Canada Book Fund.

Canada

PRINTED AND BOUND IN CANADA

ECW PRESS
ecwpress.com

CONTENTS

—

For my parents, Karen and Ron MacPherson, my husband, Chris, and our children, Ben and Sophie. For everything.
— Rhonda Church

For my parents, Elliott and Shirley MacKinnon, my wife, Leanne, and our children, Breagh, Ashlynn, and Kaylee. For all the current and future users of the Canadian health-care system.
— Neil MacKinnon

FOREWORD

◼

By John G. Abbott, B.A., M.A.

There are many "how to" books for the Canadian consumer, but this one — written for users of our universal, public health-care system — is long overdue. Shouldn't we already have a manual to help guide us through the crucial process of managing our own health? How often have we returned from a visit to the family doctor or a specialist only to find we forgot to ask that one significant question about our care? While we trust our health-care providers, what is our role? Isn't the onus on us to take some control over our own health and our encounters with the health-care delivery system, beginning with the initial office visit to our family doctor, the gateway to our medical care?

An important component of primary health care is self-management: when a patient participates in — or educates themselves about — their own treatment. The more information we have about our own health and the care we receive, the more we become involved, the better our health outcomes. The Health Council of Canada has released several reports on the role primary health care plays in our health-care system. We recognize that the family physician and other health-care providers are pivotal players in our care. With more Canadians developing one or more chronic health conditions, we have come to rely more heavily on our health system. But is this what we really want? Shouldn't we want, instead, more information about our disease? More knowledge of what we can do to prevent and/or manage it without total reliance on (read abdication to) our health-care system? And, once we engage the health-care system, do we have the understanding to engage as true partners in our own care?

The beauty and real contribution of *Take as Directed* is that the authors understand the importance of the patient being an informed and equal participant in his or her own care and that each encounter should benefit both the patient and the provider.

As a health-care policy specialist, I examine whether our public policies and programs — often promoted with much fanfare — resonate with Canadians. One way to assess these solutions is to see how clearly the messages are written and understood, with the most successful being written with the patient in mind. This book will succeed where others have failed for just that reason. We can now do our homework before our next trip to the doctor's office.

John G. Abbott is currently chief executive officer with the Health Council of Canada. In addition, he is a management consultant with the Institute for the Advancement of Public Policy, a private consulting firm specializing in public policy analysis and development. Abbott has held a number of senior positions with the Newfoundland and Labrador government, including serving as deputy minister of health and community services, where he oversaw the reorganization of the province's system of regional health authorities and the expansion of the provincial drug program. He was recognized in 1999 with the Lieutenant Governor's Award for Excellence in Public Administration by the Institute for Public Administration of Canada.

CHAPTER ONE

PAUL'S
PERIL

A Cautionary Tale

Before Paul's wife, Katharine, left to go shopping in the city earlier this morning, she gave him explicit instructions. "Go get an antibiotic for that cold. You don't want it to get any worse and spoil our cruise. And I don't want to catch it." She left their family doctor's phone number on the kitchen table beside his breakfast and his morning pills.

Both former teachers, Paul and Katharine had retired a few months earlier. After perusing an array of glossy brochures, they settled on a cruise of the Greek Islands to celebrate the beginning of this exciting phase in their lives. They were to leave in six days and visit their daughter in London, England, before flying on to Athens.

"Don't let the doctor give you one of those old-fashioned penicillins," Katharine told Paul as she kissed him goodbye. "They never work. Get something strong."

Paul heads to the local emergency department after learning that his family doctor is away until the following week. The waiting room is chockablock with people who are coughing, cuddling runny-nosed babies, limping on twisted ankles, and pressing damp face cloths to skin lacerations in need of repair. A number of ambulances arrive during the almost two hours that Paul waits.

When Paul is finally seen by the harried young physician, he explains that he woke up with a cold yesterday, that he and his wife are soon leaving on a cruise, and that she insisted he get an antibiotic so he isn't sick while they are travelling. He answers the doctor's questions: No, he doesn't have a fever. He's not coughing anything up. He had a sore throat, but it's going away — it's mostly just a head cold.

Paul went over his background health with the triage nurse earlier, but the doctor asks similar questions. Paul has had diabetes for the last six years, he explains. He was admitted to hospital about a year and a half ago with angina. He's on a few medications. He knows one is Aspirin, and he thinks one is for his blood pressure and one for his diabetes. No, he tells the doctor, he doesn't know their names. One is blue and white and one is a peachy colour. There's another one, a little white one, but he's not sure what it is or what it's for. His wife looks after all his medications — he just takes what she leaves out for him.

The doctor examines him. "It looks like a virus," he says. "The best thing is to wait it out. Drink fluids and get lots of rest."

"I've been waiting here for almost two hours. Can't you just give me an antibiotic? It's not like I take them all the time."

The doctor looks at Paul. "Antibiotics only kill bacteria. They don't kill viruses. It's really not going to help you. You'll be feeling much better in about three days, even without an antibiotic."

"Can't you give me a prescription in case I don't feel better in a few days? I don't want to have to come back again — or to have to find a doctor in Greece."

The doctor hesitates but finally agrees. "Just promise me you'll wait a few days before you start taking it. If you're feeling better, just toss the prescription out."

"One more thing," Paul tells the doctor. "My wife wants me to get something stronger than penicillin."

The doctor shrugs and scribbles out a prescription. He passes it to Paul as the sound of an ambulance siren beckons him away.

On the drive home, Paul stops at the pharmacy half a block from the hospital. He isn't sure which pharmacy Katharine uses; it does-n't cross his mind that it should matter. He tells the pharmacist the same things he told the doctor about his other medications. Paul buys a bottle of water at the front of the store and takes the first pill in the car on the way home.

Four days later Paul awakens feeling terrible. He has had a back-ache and sore shoulder muscles for a few days, but he's been blaming it on the yard work he's been doing in preparation for their time away. This morning, though, even before he gets out of bed, he feels much worse. "It's like I'm getting the flu all over again," he tells Katharine.

"It sounds like the antibiotic isn't working," Katharine says. "The doctor didn't give you penicillin, did he?"

"I asked him not to."

Paul gets out of bed with considerable difficulty. His muscles are weak and painful, which makes it difficult to stand, much less walk down the hall to the bathroom.

"I'm taking you back to the hospital. I think you need a stronger antibiotic," Katharine says.

With her help, Paul eventually manages to reach the toilet. He notices that his urine has an odd tea-coloured hue.

Katharine carries a list of their prescription medications in her wallet and she passes it to the triage nurse when they arrive at the hospital. The doctor who saw Paul four days ago is again working in the emergency department. Paul admits, somewhat sheepishly, that he began taking the antibiotic immediately after his last visit.

After an examination and a series of investigations, the doctor diag-noses rhabdomyolysis — a condition that is causing disintegration of muscle tissue throughout Paul's body. He tells Paul and Katharine the condition is very rare but is most likely due to an interaction between the antibiotic Paul is taking and one of the medications he takes at home. Unfortunately the doctor did not have access to Paul's list of medications when he saw him four days ago. He tells Paul and Katharine that rhabdomyolysis is a potentially life-threatening condition and that up to two-thirds of all individuals with this condition develop kidney failure that may require dialysis.

Paul is admitted to hospital. He develops kidney failure, but it resolves without dialysis. Nonetheless, he spends almost two weeks in hospital. After he is discharged from hospital it is many months before Paul is strong enough to return to his usual activities. The planned Greek cruise, of course, is cancelled.

Recently, much attention has been paid to the issue of errors occurring within the health-care system. A 2004 landmark study by Baker and Norton, for example, showed that one out of every thirteen (7.5%) adult patients in Canadian hospitals experienced at least one adverse event; many of these were errors related to the prescribing or administration of medication.[1]

When an individual experiences an adverse event, a number of factors come into play and ultimately culminate in the outcome. Health-care providers often use the "Swiss cheese model"[2] to explain how poor outcomes occur. At each stage of a health-care encounter, there is a risk that something could go wrong, much like a small hole in a block of Swiss cheese. Paul, for example, was at increased risk for an adverse outcome because he was unable to convey to his caregivers the names of the medications he was taking. Normally, a series of checks and balances are inherent in the delivery of health care; think of them as the substance of the cheese itself, preventing one small error, or Swiss cheese hole, from aligning with other small holes and resulting in a large hole, or a significant problem for the patient. Paul, for example, had a number of "holes" that aligned to create his unfortunate illness. Besides his lack of information about his medications, he requested a prescription for a medication that he probably did not need. He was seen by a physician who was extremely busy, unfamiliar with him, and did not have access to a list of his regular medications. Similarly, Paul's prescription was filled by a pharmacist who was unfamiliar with him and with the other medications he was taking. These all seem like minor matters, but when they align for one patient during a single health-care encounter, the outcome can be catastrophic.

Usually, of course, taking an unnecessary antibiotic does not result in a near-fatal illness. (It does, however, contribute to growing resistance to antibiotics, which will be discussed in Chapter 4.) Had Paul seen his regular family physician, she would have been aware of the other medications he was taking. Probably, she would not have prescribed the antibiotic that resulted in rhabdomyolysis when it was taken in combination with another of Paul's medications. We know that the busier a physician is, the greater the chance he or she will prescribe an unnecessary antibiotic for a common cold.[3] Had the physician seeing Paul been less busy, he might not have agreed to issue the prescription. That day, though, chances are it was faster to write the prescription than to continue to argue with Paul that he didn't need it. If the pharmacist had been familiar with Paul, she would also have had records indicating what medications Paul was taking and would have, in all likelihood, contacted Paul's physician to discuss the potential drug interaction prior to dispensing the antibiotic that made Paul ill.

Health-care providers and policy makers, as well as independent organizations such as the Canadian Patient Safety Institute, look for the root causes of adverse events and how health-care practices can be changed to make delivery of health care safer. However, each of us has a critical role to play in ensuring that we have the best possible outcome from our encounters with the Canadian health-care system, including using medications in a safe, responsible, and appropriate fashion.

In this book we will empower you to obtain the best and safest possible health-care outcome from your encounters with the Canadian health-care system and have your medication work safely and effectively for you. After a behind-the-scenes look at how our health-care system works, or doesn't work, we will draw on our experience as a family physician and a pharmacist and researcher and walk you through a visit to your doctor or to a hospital. We will tell you how to prepare for a visit to your regular physician and how to deal with an unexpected illness or injury when you are cared for by an unfamiliar provider. We will talk about situations in which the best remedy is no medication at all. In the event that medication is prescribed, we will tell you what information you shouldn't leave the doctor's clinic or the hospital without.

We will also review your encounter with the pharmacist, who dispenses your medication, and offer tips on how you can make the very best use of your pharmacist's expertise. We'll tell you how to safely use your medications at home, what to do if you believe your medication isn't working, and where you should turn if you think you're experiencing a side effect. We'll also offer tips on accessing medications if you are having difficulty affording them, where to find credible drug information on the internet, and how to decide if a nontraditional medication such as an herbal remedy is right for you.

In writing this book, we have created a number of vignettes, such as the one of Paul and Katharine, based on people we have cared for and worked with. However, in order to protect their privacy, it was necessary to mask and alter details that could identify them. In some cases, the stories we tell are based on composite patients.

First up — let's examine just how safe our health-care system is, or isn't, and look at what factors contribute to an optimum health-care outcome for you.

◉

CHAPTER TWO

HEALTH-CARE
SAFETY

An Oxymoron?

In *Take as Directed*, we will walk you through the various steps of the health-care system to help you get the most out of your health-care experience. Throughout the book, we will have a special focus on medications but much of the advice and perspective we bring will be applicable beyond just your use of prescription and over-the-counter drugs. Before we begin this journey through the various professions, settings, and locations of our health-care system, however, we will address in the next two chapters some of the "big picture" issues of our health-care system. The first of these issues is the safety, or lack thereof, of our health-care system and medication use.

What's in a Name?

Many words and phrases describe adverse consequences of health care and, more specifically, of medications. A few of the more commonly used terms include *adverse drug events, adverse drug reactions, drug-related morbidity, medication errors, medication incidents, medication misadventures,* and *side effects.* These terms are often used interchangeably, even though they can mean quite different

---

things. Phrases such as *medical error* and *medication error* also can convey a sense of blame. Unfortunately, even experts in the field misuse terms on occasion and sometimes cannot agree on which terms should be used. Some experts in Canada tried to bring some clarity to this issue a few years ago by creating a publication called the *Canadian Patient Safety Dictionary*. So, what is one to do to survive these potentially confusing terms?

In *Take as Directed*, we will primarily be using the terms *adverse events (AEs) and* adverse drug events *(ADEs)*. These are well-recognized terms that were used in the largest study of adverse health-care consequences in Canada to date. As defined by the *Canadian Patient Safety Dictionary*, an adverse event is "an unexpected and undesired incident directly associated with care or services provided to a patient; an incident that occurs during the process of providing health care and that results in patient injury or death; an adverse outcome for a patient, including injury or complication."[4]

There will be some exceptions to our use of these two terms. Most of these exceptions involve reporting the results of studies where a different term, medical error, was used. While we personally would not have chosen to use that term, we need to use it within the context discussing the results of those studies to avoid distorting the meaning of the study results.

Oprah Winfrey and Health-Care System Adverse Events

Due to Oprah Winfrey's popularity and cultural influence, when she pays attention to a new book, movie, or issue, there is often a ripple effect throughout the United States, Canada, and beyond as others start to pay attention to that same issue. For an author, having your book endorsed by Oprah is almost a guarantee that you will be on a bestseller list. At times, Oprah has appeared on lists of the most influential celebrities and women around the world.

So, when Oprah devoted an entire episode of her TV program, *The Oprah Winfrey Show*, on March 10, 2009, to adverse events, a lot of people started to think seriously about this issue. She interviewed Hollywood actor Dennis Quaid and his wife, Kimberly, about a serious adverse drug event that almost claimed the lives of their newborn twins (see "Dennis Quaid and Deadly Heparin"). She included many other real-life tales of adverse events, including a mother who discovered that she didn't have breast cancer until after having a mastectomy.

Dennis Quaid and Deadly Heparin

It was a time of joy. Hollywood actor Dennis Quaid and his wife, Kimberly, had welcomed their newborn twins, Thomas Boone and Zoe Grace, just two weeks earlier. The twins were doing well but had remained in hospital.

Then everything changed as the Quaids were told that their twins had been two of three infants at Cedars-Sinai Medical Center in Los Angeles who had experienced an adverse drug event. All three infants had been given an injection of a drug called heparin, which is used to thin blood and prevent clots. Instead of receiving the typical dose for infants of 10 units, the babies each received a dose of 10,000 units. As a result of receiving 1,000 times the typical dose of heparin, the newborns started to bleed internally. Although the twins ultimately survived after spending several days in the neonatal intensive care unit, the Quaids reached a settlement of U.S.$750,000 with the hospital and the hospital was fined by the California Department of Public Health.

Unfortunately, this was not the first such error involving an overdose of heparin. Moreover, other similar events have happened since the episode involving the Quaids' newborn twins. As a result of their experience and other similar errors, the Quaids have become public advocates for improving health-care safety and preventing adverse drug events. In addition to TV appearances on shows such as *60 Minutes*

---

and *The Oprah Winfrey Show*, Dennis Quaid often speaks to front-line health professionals. For example, he gave the keynote address at the American Society of Health-System Pharmacists Midyear Clinical Meeting in Las Vegas in December 2009.

In our country, the Institute for Safe Medication Practices Canada has been actively educating health-care professionals about how to prevent these events, such as developing a heparin tool kit. Accreditation Canada, which accredits our hospitals, has introduced new recommendations about using heparin in patient care areas of hospitals.[5] Even the World Health Organization has recognized the seriousness of this issue, creating a new initiative called *Action on Patient Safety: High 5s*, which includes strategies for dealing with high-concentration IV drugs. We hope these efforts will help prevent other parents from experiencing the type of agonizing situation experienced by the Quaids.

Was Oprah onto something, or were these stories of adverse events simply a way to boost TV ratings? Are there real, trustworthy statistics to support the attention given to this issue? How does the safety of the health-care system in Canada compare to other similar countries? What are the factors that place an individual at risk for experiencing an adverse event? How common are adverse drug events? These are some of the questions we will answer in this chapter.

Is the Health-Care System Safe?

We probably don't need to state the obvious, but we will anyway — the health-care system is very complex. There are untold combinations of interactions each day between different types of health professionals (physicians, pharmacists, nurses, occupational therapists, etc.), working in different types of settings (physician offices, pharmacies, hospitals, long-term care facilities, private clinics, etc.), dealing with different types of clinical problems and diseases (cancer, diabetes, asthma, etc.), using different types of strategies to deal with these problems (medications, surgery, laboratory tests, etc.). A diagram trying to capture all these interactions would quickly become an ugly mess.

A second obvious statement is that there is considerable risk in health care. Patients respond differently to the same medication or surgical procedure. Often a clear and concise diagnosis cannot be made, and thus physicians and other clinicians are faced with making difficult choices under conditions of uncertainly. There is an inherent risk in any health-care intervention — whether the intervention is a medication, surgery, or diagnostic procedure. One solution to reducing health-care adverse events that would be absurd but effective is to stop health-care interventions altogether.

Given that we cannot or would not want to stop all health-care interventions, a more useful task is to figure out how often adverse events occur in health care, why they occur, and then to develop strategies to reduce these events.

As we have just stated, health care is a system associated with high risk. This, however, is not a "cop-out" for health care that makes adverse events excusable. In fact, there are many other high-risk systems that have succeeded in improving safety and reducing harm to others. The following table compares health care to several of these systems, such as road safety, commercial aviation, and the nuclear industry. As one can see from quickly scanning this table, health care does not compare favourably to these other systems and is similar in risk to mountain climbing. Whereas mountain climbing is a risk that its participants freely choose, users of the health-care system rarely participate by choice but rather have been forced to use the system because they or a family member has received a sudden and unpleasant diagnosis, or has been in an accident.

Comparing the Safety of Health Care to Other Systems[6]

Nature of System	Risk of Unintended Incidents	Examples	Typical Safety Measures
Dangerous (very unsafe)	Greater than 10^{-3} (1 in 1,000)	Mountain climbing; much of health care	System relies on regulation of individual performance
Regulated systems	Between 10^{-3} and 10^{-5} (1 in 1,000 and 1 in 100,000)	Road safety; chemical industry; chartered airlines; anesthesia for low-risk patients; gastroenterologic endoscopy	System uses regulations and procedures to govern performance; focuses on error-resistant design of work, on standardization, and on limits to professional autonomy
Ultra-safe systems	10^{-6} and safer (1 in 1,000,000)	Commercial aviation; European railroads; nuclear industry; blood transfusion	Priority given to safety rather than performance improvement; highly regulated limits on action by individual performers

Is the Health-Care System in Canada Safe?

Prior to 2004, we couldn't really answer the question "Is the health-care system in Canada safe?" Some small studies showed problems in certain areas, but no large study could truly give us a comprehensive picture of patient safety in health care. This changed in 2004, when the first large national study of adverse events was published in the *Canadian Medical Association Journal*. "The Canadian Adverse Events Study" involved researchers reviewing the medical charts of more than 3,700 Canadians. They discovered an alarming trend: 7.5% of the adult hospital patients they reviewed had unintended adverse events during their hospitalization. The percentage may seem low, but when one considers the large number of Canadians who are hospitalized in any given year, this percentage extrapolates to approximately 185,000 adverse events in hospitalized adult Canadians each year. The researchers observed that the adverse events often led to other problems, such as an extension of the hospital stay, injury to the patient, and in some cases even death. Almost 40% of these incidents were judged to be preventable. [7] The authors of this study later commented that the trends they observed in Canada were similar to the experience in comparable nations such as the United States, the United Kingdom, Australia, and New Zealand.[8]

One area that seems to be especially problematic in health care is the transfer of patient care from one health professional to another (e.g., from a family physician to a medical specialist) or one institution to another (e.g., from a hospital to a long-term care facility). While ideally we'd like to have seamless health care where the patient's relevant information is transferred easily, often this does not occur. As a result, there is a great opportunity for error during these transitions in care.

Two studies have documented error during transitions of care in Canada. In the first study, conducted at a hospital in Ottawa, patients were followed after being discharged from hospital to see whether they developed an adverse event. Within just fourteen weeks' post-discharge from hospital, almost one in four (23%) patients developed an adverse event. Medications were involved in almost three of every four (72%) adverse events, or in about 17% of all patients who were discharged from the hospital.[9]

In the second study, conducted in Moncton, New Brunswick, a hospital pharmacist conducted an in-depth review of the patients' medications just prior to discharge from the hospital. The pharmacist found, on average, 3.5 drug-related problems per patient in the study. Approximately one in three of these problems involved a situation where the patient was about to be discharged from the hospital even though he or she should have received additional drug therapy. When reviewed by other health professionals, about three-quarters of the problems were deemed to be significant or very significant.[10]

Do Canadians Believe Their Health-Care System Is Safe?

We have just reviewed some of the research about health-care adverse events in Canada. However, is this a topic of concern to just a small group of researchers? What do Canadians in general think about this topic and how does their perception compare to those in similar nations?

One organization that can help us answer this question is the Commonwealth Fund, a private foundation based in New York City. Its goal is to promote a high-performing health-care system in the United States. One method it uses to try to accomplish this goal is to look at health-care approaches in other western, industrialized countries and apply lessons it learns to the United States.

Each year the Commonwealth Fund conducts an international survey of health-care practice and policy. The questions and target audience differ from year to year. Its 2007 survey captured the perspective of 12,000 adults in seven countries (Australia, Canada, Germany, the Netherlands, New Zealand, the United Kingdom, and the United States). Slightly more than 3,000 adult Canadians were included in this survey. The survey addressed a wide variety of questions related to the health-care experience of these individuals, ranging from health-care costs to access, quality, and safety.[11]

The following table contains the results from three questions that were asked about adverse events. Overall, about one in six Canadians said they had personally experienced a medical, medication, or laboratory error in the previous two years. Using data from the 2006 census, this would extrapolate to about 4.2 million Canadians (17% of 24.7 million adults Canadians) who said they have experienced at least one health-care error in the past two years.[12] Another way of looking at this number would be to say that a number equivalent to the entire population of Saskatchewan, Manitoba, the three Maritime provinces, and the three territories experiences at least one health-care error every two years. That sentence should cause all Canadians to reflect on the safety of our health-care system.

Every study has its limitations, as does this survey. Individuals who gave these responses over the course of a telephone interview were giving their own perspective on this issue (i.e., self-reporting) and their responses have not been validated with other research methods such as medical chart reviews that were part of the "Canadian Adverse Events Study." Still, the continuity of the responses among the seven countries included in the survey does lend credibility to the results. It is worth noting that Canada placed third worst in overall self-reported medical error rate.

Self-Reported Medical Error in Canada and in Six Other Nations[13]

Percentage of surveyed patients who reported errors in past two years	Australia	Canada	Germany	The Netherlands	New Zealand	United Kingdom	United States
Experienced medical or medication error	15	10	9	9	11	9	13
Experienced lab or diagnostic test error	11	12	4	8	9	10	14
Experienced any medical, medication, or lab error	20	17	12	14	16	13	20

If you are interested in learning more about patient safety, including issues related to medications, visit the following websites.

Canadian Patient Safety Institute (CPSI)
www.patientsafetyinstitute.ca

Families Launching Action Against Medication Errors www.flaame.org

Institute for Safe Medication Practices (ISMP) Canada
www.safemedicationuse.ca

MedEffect Canada (Health Canada)
www.hc-sc.gc.ca/dhp-mps/medeff/index-eng.php

World Health Organization (WHO) Patients for Patient Safety
www.who.int/patientsafety/patients_for_patient/en/

The SafetyNET-Rx Research Project www.safetynetrx.ca

How Do Patient Perceptions Compare to Health Professional Perceptions?

You may be wondering how the perceptions of patients compare to the perceptions of health-care professionals such as physicians, nurses, pharmacists, and managers. Are our nation's health-care workers concerned about the issue of adverse events? A survey published in 2006 provides some insight into this question. The respondents were asked, "Are you likely to be subject to a serious medical error while treated in a Canadian hospital?" Sixty percent of the public who were asked this question replied that it was "likely" that they would be subject to such an error. The response of the pharmacists in the survey was the closest to the public response, with 62% of pharmacists saying it was "likely" that someone would be subject to such an error. Nurses (74%) and managers (77%) thought it was "very likely" that someone would be subject to such an error, while physicians (40%) were less convinced. So, this survey confirms that patient perceptions on the issue of error are not out of line with the perceptions of health-care professionals.[14]

What Places an Individual at Risk for a Medical Error?

Thus far, this chapter may seem rather depressing. We have reviewed the issue of health-care safety from a variety of perspectives and evidence that strongly suggests there is a significant problem related to the lack of a safe health-care system. Our intent is not to sound alarmist and say the "sky is falling," but we do want to ensure that you are aware of the seriousness of this issue.

That being said, one of our goals in writing *Take as Directed* is to empower you so that you can avoid adverse outcomes and get the most out of your health-care experience. One way to do this is to determine whether you are personally at risk for experiencing a medical error. We will be using the results of a recent study to help you assess your own risk.

"Self-Reported Medical Errors in Seven Countries: Implications for Canada" was published in 2009 in the main patient safety scientific journal in Canada, *Patient Safety Papers*.[15] This journal is published once a year and typically contains some of the most interesting and innovative research on patient safety in our country. One of the co-authors of this paper is a co-author of this book (NM), so we can share some special insights that did not appear in the published study. The study used data from the 2007 Commonwealth Fund international health-care survey, which comes from the perspective of individuals living in these seven countries, not from the perspective of health-care professionals or other health-care decision-makers. The term *medical error* was used in study and so we will also use that phrase when discussing the results, although as we previously stated, we would have preferred the term *adverse event*.

The study used an advanced statistical technique in order to determine what distinguishes the 1,938 patients in the survey who said they had personally experienced at least one medical error in the past two years from the 7,652 patients who did not experience an error. The study looked at differences in patient demographics (gender, age, etc.), access to care, coordination of care, and the patient/health-care professional relationship. In the final analysis, there were seven risk factors for self-reported medical errors, as shown in the following table.

Risk Factors for Self-Reported Medical Error[16]

Lack of patient involvement in care
Perceived inadequate nursing staffing
Absence of a regular doctor
Use of 4+ medications
Age under 65
Lack of physician time with patient
Presence of a chronic condition

One way to think about these risk factors is as your own personal checklist to gauge your risk of experiencing a medical error in the future. Of course, even if none of the seven risk factors applies to you, it does not mean that you have no risk at all for experiencing a medical error in the future; it simply means you have a lower risk.

1. Lack of patient involvement in care

Of all seven risk factors identified in this study, this first one — lack of patient involvement in care — had the strongest relationship with self-reported adverse event. In fact, patients who replied "no" to the question "Were you involved as much as you wanted to be in decisions about your care and treatment?" were about twice as likely to have experienced a medical error as those who responded "yes." So, if there is just one thing to remember from this chapter, it is this message: Be proactive in your own health-care experience. You will find this is an ongoing theme in *Take as Directed*, as we provide a variety of checklists, tools, websites, and other resources to empower you in your own care or those of your loved ones. This is not simply about becoming more confident or increasing your knowledge of your conditions and medications. As this study suggests, there are serious consequences when you are not involved in your own care.

2. Perceived inadequate nursing staffing

When health care works best, it is a team approach with contributions from a wide range of health professionals and staff in addition to physicians. Nurses, in particular, are often singled out by patients for their caring and empathy. In the Commonwealth Fund study, patients who had been hospitalized at least once in the previous two years were asked, "In your opinion, were there always or nearly always enough nurses to care for you during your hospital stay?" Those who answered "no" were almost 1.8 times as likely to have experienced a medical error as those who responded "yes." Of course, no researcher checked into the staffing levels of nurses in the hospitals on the days in which these patients were hospitalized so we have to take these responses at their face value. Still, as patients who have been hospitalized will readily attest, even lying in a hospital bed, one can quickly recognize if nurses are stressed and stretched to the maximum. In Canada, we know that there is a current shortage of nurses and frequent burnout among hospital nurses who are working in difficult environments. Ensuring that we have sufficient numbers of nurses in our hospitals should not only be an issue for our nursing unions but for every Canadian.

3. Absence of a regular doctor

In addition to a shortage of nurses and other allied health professionals such as pharmacists, there is a shortage of family physicians in Canada. In the next chapter, we will examine this issue in detail. Here, we will address this issue in the context of patient safety. In this study, patients who said they did not have a regular doctor were almost twice as likely to have experienced a medical error. In a later chapter, we will review the concept of a *medical home*; that is, having a regular doctor not in name only but being able to access him or her when you need to and having that person coordinate your whole care. In another recently published study that also used data from the Commonwealth Fund international survey, more than half (51%) of adult Canadians surveyed did not have a medical home.[17] Canadians who did not have a medical home were both more likely to have experienced a medical error and a medication error. So, while Canadians are familiar with the old adage "an apple a day keeps the doctor away," a new saying that is particularly relevant in light of this new data is "access to a regular doctor helps keeps errors away."

4. Use of four or more medications
In the survey, about one out of every four patients who used four or more medications experienced a medical error. This is roughly a 30% increase in the error rate over those who use three or fewer medications. One key message here is that these medications included all types of drugs: prescription and over-the-counter medications, herbal products, and others. As we will review in a later chapter, having a complete record of all the medications you take is critical as there can be significant interactions among them. Later in this chapter, we will review medications that are strongly associated with harm and/or death.

5. Age under sixty-five
This is the one risk factor that was a surprise to the study investigators. Heading into the study, they expected to find seniors to be at a greater risk for reporting medical error, but in fact the opposite was discovered. There could be several reasons to help explain this somewhat perplexing result. Seniors may be less willing to question their physician and other health-care providers about possible errors and thus less likely to report errors as well. Many seniors grew up in a time

when questioning the judgment of your physician was not viewed to be proper behaviour and one was more accepting of a physician's advice. Secondly, as the amount of post-secondary education has increased in recent decades, perhaps adults younger than sixty-five, who in general have more education, may be more willing to research their health-care condition and treatment and thus pick up on potential errors. Regardless of what is the real explanation, medical errors can happen to anyone no matter their age, as almost one in five seniors in this study said they had experienced a medical error.

6. Lack of physician time with patient

Admittedly, some Canadians do not like doctor visits and their main goal is to get in and out as fast as they can. However, many other Canadians feel rushed during visits and wish they had more time to ask their doctor questions. This study has shown that there are severe consequences to rushed doctor visits. Patients who responded "rarely" or "no" when asked, "When you need care or treatment, does your general practitioner/regular doctor/the doctor explain things in a way you can understand?" were almost 1.7 times as likely to have experienced a medical error. We feel strongly about maximizing the interaction of a patient-physician visit and thus have allocated an entire chapter in *Take as Directed* to preparing for your visits and another chapter to the visit itself.

7. Presence of a chronic condition

The final risk factor for self-reported medical error in the study was presence of at least one chronic condition, such as diabetes, asthma, or high blood pressure. Of the Canadians in the study, 17% reported having experienced an error if they had one chronic condition. This increased to 28% among Canadians who had two or more chronic conditions.

We hope this detailed look at risk factors for medical error has caused you to reflect on your own status and risk for error. Of course, some of these risk factors can be changed while others, such as age and presence of a chronic condition, are not within our control. Now that we have reviewed trends and risk factors for medical error, we will focus specifically on medication use.

Medication Use in Canada

For many Canadians, medications are a key part of their health-care experience. Prescription and non-prescription drugs help millions of Canadians by improving quality of life, curing disease, and reducing the signs and symptoms of disease. We may take the availability of medications for granted, however; it was not too long ago that most of the medications in use today did not exist. Conditions such as scarlet fever that were at one time associated with considerable morbidity and mortality are now readily treatable with the right medications. Even in the last number of years, the treatment for many stomach and intestinal ulcers has moved from surgery to a simple regimen of prescription drugs taken over a short duration of time. Simply put, medications are one of the greatest tools available today in modern medicine.

At the same time, we know that outcomes from medication use are not always optimal. There is considerable evidence that medications are often overused, underused, or inappropriately used. Each drug has its own side-effect profile and often adverse drug events result, harming patients. There are also risks with the use of medications that are preventable, and recent research has indicated that these types of preventable events injure a significant number of Canadians.

Finally, the cost of medications is a real concern for both individual Canadians who may have to spend their own money on prescriptions and for health-care payers such as provincial governments. The following table reviews some of the issues related to prescription drug access, affordability, quality, and safety, and shows how Canada compares to other nations.

International Comparisons on Prescription Access, Affordability, Quality, and Safety[4]

	Canada	Australia	Germany	The Netherlands	New Zealand	United Kingdom	United States
Health-care overview							
Comprehensive national minimum health insurance benefits package	Yes	Yes	Yes	Yes	Yes	Yes	No
Prescription drugs are included as a core benefit	No	Yes	Yes	Yes	Yes	Yes	No
The perspective of primary-care physicians							
Routinely uses electronic prescribing of medications	11%	81%	59%	85%	78%	55%	20%
Routinely receives alert or complaint about a potential problem with drug dose or interaction using a computerized system	10%	80%	40%	93%	87%	91%	23%
Easily generates list of medications taken by patients, including Rxs by other doctors	25%	74%	55%	59%	72%	88%	37%

	Canada	Australia	Germany	The Netherlands	New Zealand	United Kingdom	United States
The perspective of primary-care physicians (continued)							
Believes that their patients often experience difficulty paying for prescriptions	24%	15%	23%	7%	27%	13%	51%
Practice has a documented process for follow-up and analysis of all adverse events (including adverse drug events)	20%	35%	32%	7%	41%	79%	37%
The perspective of adults							
Confident they receive the most effective drugs	32%	36%	23%	45%	20%	25%	33%
Spent $500 or more out of pocket for prescriptions in the past year (for those regularly taking prescriptions)	27%	30%	10%	1%	13%	2%	42%

	Canada	Australia	Germany	The Netherlands	New Zealand	United Kingdom	United States
The perspective of adults with chronic conditions							
In the past two years, did not fill prescription or skipped doses because of cost	18%	20%	12%	3%	18%	7%	43%
In the past two years, was given the wrong medication or wrong dose	10%	13%	7%	6%	13%	9%	14%

Spending on Medications

Total spending on prescription and non-prescription drugs in Canada rose from $21.8 billion in 2004 to $30 billion in 2009, an increase of 37% during this time period.[19] Pharmaceuticals are now the second single-largest category of health-care expenses in Canada, trailing only hospitals. Prescription drugs account for 14% of total health-care spending in our country, although there are considerable differences across the country, as can be seen in "Spending on Prescription Drugs." Moreover, as "Overall Spending on Prescription Drugs by Age Group" and "Overall Spending on Prescription Drugs by Province and Age Group" demonstrate, there are also considerable differences according to age category, with seniors consuming far more medications than the other age groups.

So what is driving this spending increase? Dr. Steve Morgan and colleagues at the University of British Columbia have studied the trends in spending on drugs and have attempted to determine what is driving the changes. As one might suspect, increasing overall life expectancy as well as an aging population are driving some of the increase as baby boomers start to enter an age where their use of prescription medications increases and as overall life expectancy in Canada increases. The average cost per prescription is also partially responsible for the increase. A third factor driving costs is what Morgan and his colleagues call "therapeutic choice effects," meaning that prescribers are choosing more costly medications over less costly ones when prescribing. However, the major driver of the increase in spending on drugs is an increase in the volume of prescriptions.[20] Simply put, more prescriptions are being filled than ever before in our country.

Spending on Prescription Drugs[21]

Percentage of health-care spending accounted for by perscription drugs, 2007

Source: Canadian Rx Atlas, 2nd Ed. Data from the Canadian Institute for Health Information, Drug Expenditure in Canada, 1985–2007. No data available for Northern Canada.

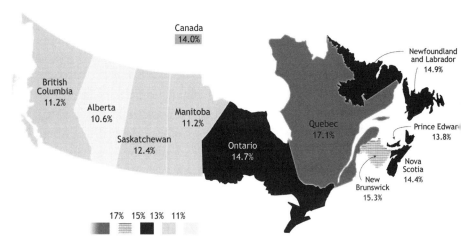

Overall Spending on Prescription Drugs by Age Group[22]
Per capita spending in Canada by age group, 2007
Source: Canadian Rx Atlas, 2nd Ed.

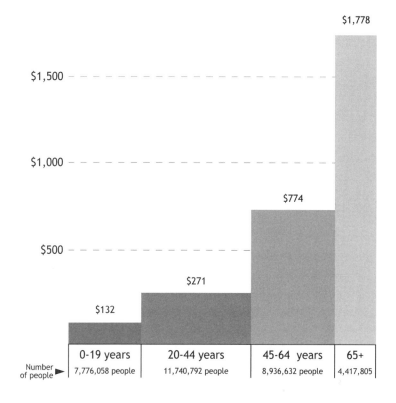

	0-19 years	20-44 years	45-64 years	65+
	$132	$271	$774	$1,778
Number of people ►	7,776,058 people	11,740,792 people	8,936,632 people	4,417,805

Overall Spending on Prescription Drugs by Province and Age Group[23]
Per capita spending by province and age group, 2007
Source: Canadian Rx Atlas, 2nd Ed.

All Ages

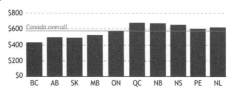

Ages 0–19

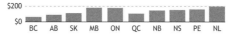

Ages 20–44

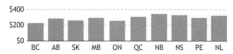

Ages 45–64

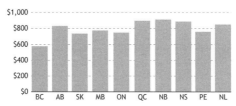

Ages 65+

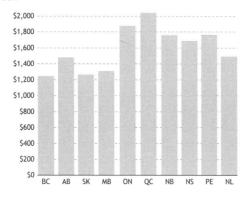

Access to Medications

Not surprisingly, as spending on drugs increases at a rate well above the general inflation rate, those who pay for drugs — governments, private payers such as employers, and Canadians — are struggling with issues related to affordability. "Degrees of Access to Drugs" shows how decisions to provide no access, partial access, or full access to a drug by a third-party payer, such as a provincial drug plan, impacts the drug and the patient involved. What may be surprising to some Canadians is how widely provincial drug plans vary in the number of drugs for which they provide coverage (see "Coverage of Medications by Provincial Drug Formularies"). It may also surprise many Canadians to know of the difference in drug coverage decisions for our politicians and bureaucrats as compared to the general public (see "Do Politicians Have Better Drug Coverage Than Average Canadians?"). In our next chapter, we will pick up on this theme and address issues related to drug policy in our country, including catastrophic drug coverage.

Degrees of Access to Drugs[24]

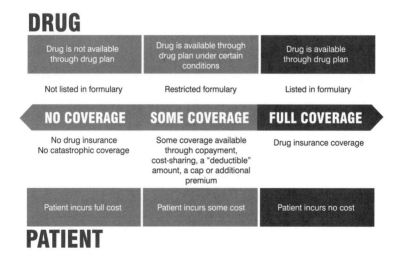

DRUG

Drug is not available through drug plan	Drug is available through drug plan under certain conditions	Drug is available through drug plan
Not listed in formulary	Restricted formulary	Listed in formulary

NO COVERAGE — **SOME COVERAGE** — **FULL COVERAGE**

No drug insurance No catastrophic coverage	Some coverage available through copayment, cost-sharing, a "deductible" amount, a cap or additional premium	Drug insurance coverage
Patient incurs full cost	Patient incurs some cost	Patient incurs no cost

PATIENT

Coverage of Medications by Provincial Drug Formularies[25]

Overall Spending
Percentage of drugs and their market value listed on provincial formularies
Source: Canadian Rx Atlas, 2nd Ed.

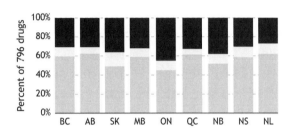

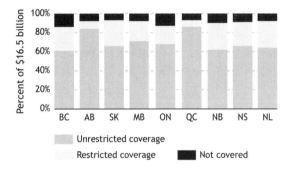

Unrestricted coverage

Restricted coverage   ■ Not covered

Do Politicians Have Better Drug Coverage Than Average Canadians?
A study released in 2007 by CARP (Canada's Association for the Fifty Plus) compared prescription drug coverage for elected and public officials to public drug plans in three provinces — Alberta, British Columbia, and Ontario — and those managed by the federal government for Canadian Aboriginals, veterans, and soldiers. The study showed a large discrepancy between the universal drug coverage enjoyed by politicians and bureaucrats and the public drug plans in several jurisdictions. These discrepancies existed for drugs that were recommended to be listed in provincial drug plans, drugs that were

recommended not to be listed, and for those drugs still waiting a recommendation by the national organization that makes such
recommendations, the Common Drug Review (CDR). For example, of
twenty-five drugs that the CDR recommended not be listed in provincial drug plans, all twenty-five are covered by drug plans for the
federal members of Parliament and bureaucrats, while soldiers and
Aboriginals are only reimbursed for three of the twenty-five drugs.[26]

The Medication-Use System

The various steps and stages associated with Canadians' encounters
with medications can be referred to as the *medication-use system*. This
includes everything from being diagnosed with a condition that
requires medication use, to being prescribed a medication, to receiving
a medication and appropriate counselling, to ongoing monitoring to
ensure that the intended outcomes from that drug's use are being
achieved. This system also includes all the organizations such as hospitals and pharmacies and all the individuals such as physicians,
pharmacists, and pharmacy technicians involved in each step. As
many Canadians would readily recognize, this system is very complex. For example, consider the large number of diagnoses that may
involve medications in their treatment and the wide variety of medications behind the pharmacist's counter in the average community
pharmacy.

It has been argued that in order for the medication-use system to
perform in an optimal manner, eight essential elements, or components, must be present for each patient (see "Eight Elements of a
Safe and Effective Medication-Use System"). When even one of these
elements is missing for one medication for a single patient, that
patient is placed at a higher risk of experiencing an adverse drug
event. For example, while the patient's diagnosis may be correct, the
right drug may be prescribed to treat the condition, the patient may
be able to afford to purchase the medication, and the pharmacist dispenses it correctly, if the patient does not receive the properly tailored

counselling on how to take the medication, a suboptimal outcome may result. Unfortunately, the evidence suggests that at least one of the eight essential elements of a safe and effective medication-use system is missing for most patients. Thus, these eight elements should not be viewed as optional components that are sometimes in place but rather basic aspects of care that should be present for all Canadians.

Eight Elements of a Safe and Effective Medication-Use System[27]

Element	Comments
1. Timely recognition of drug indications and other signs and symptoms relevant to drug use, along with accurate identification of underlying disease.	"Correct" therapy for a late or incorrect diagnosis cannot improve a patient's quality of life.
2. Safe, accessible, and cost-effective medicines.	Safe and cost-effective (efficient) drug products must be legally and financially available.
3. Appropriate prescribing for explicit (clear, measurable, and communicable) objectives.	Explicit therapeutic objectives simplify the assessment of prescribing appropriateness and are necessary for assessing (monitoring) therapeutic outcomes.
4. Distribution, dispensing, and administration of drug products with appropriate patient advice.	This element encompasses ensuring that the patient has actually obtained the medicine, negotiating a regimen that the patient can tolerate and afford, ensuring that the patient (or caregiver) can correctly use the medicine and administration devices, and providing advice to empower the patient or caregiver to co-operate in his or her own care as much as possible.

Element	Comments
5. Participation of patients in their own care (intelligent adherence).	The ambulatory patient or caregiver should consent to therapeutic objectives and should know the signs of therapeutic success, side effects, and toxic effects; when to expect them; and what to do if they appear.
6. Monitoring (detection and resolution of problems).	Many problems can be detected before they become adverse outcomes or treatment failures.
7. Documentation and communication of information and decisions.	Documentation and communication are necessary for co-operation in a system.
8. Evaluation and improvement of products and system performance.	Practice guidelines, performance indicators, and databases are useful tools for achieving and maintaining improved system performance (outcomes).

Interacting systems

The medication-use system is just one of several systems operating within the broader health-care system. For example, there is an entire system related to laboratory tests: how these tests are ordered, performed, and reported. Moreover, medications do not act in isolation from the rest of the health-care system, but rather they often have a dramatic impact elsewhere. Research tells us that a significant percentage of all emergency department visits and hospitalizations are drug-related and many of these encounters are preventable. On the other hand, medications can reduce or prevent emergency department visits and hospitalizations. Each dollar spent on drugs by Canadians or governments is a dollar less that could be spent elsewhere. Yet, at the same time, choosing to spend money on pharmaceuticals will often reduce costs elsewhere in the health-care system.

The safety of the medication-use system
Ensuring quality care and patient safety are essential aspects of health care. One area where both of these aspects can be improved is the medication-use system. As we have previously described, the medication-use system is very complex with many different steps and individuals involved with each step. While problems can occur at any stage, we will highlight one small area — prescribing — to demonstrate the types of problems that can occur.

Each time you see a physician, whether it is within or outside the hospital setting, one of four prescribing outcomes can occur, as shown in "The Prescribing Matrix." This matrix shows the relationship of whether a prescription is indicated (needed) for a medical reason to whether a prescription was written by your prescriber during this encounter. Quadrant IV (prescription not needed and not written) does not result in problems with medication use; however, all three remaining quadrants can result in problems. One may think that Quadrant I would always result in an optimal patient outcome as in this scenario a prescription is needed and one is written. But even in Quadrant I, problems can result if clear, measurable, and communicable prescribing objectives are not known and understood by the physician, the pharmacist, and yourself. In addition, we know from studies that many patients experience a suboptimal outcome even if they were prescribed the correct medication at the correct dose, and so on. Many patients experience side effects or adverse drug reactions with medications or the medication may simply fail to achieve the desired outcome (i.e., it doesn't do what it was intended to do). Patients in Quadrants II and III are in danger of experiencing problems. In Quadrant II, the patient receives a medication they simply do not need. Many studies conducted in Canada and beyond have concluded that this type of scenario occurs quite commonly, especially with certain types of drugs such as benzodiazepines (often given to sedate patients). In Quadrant III, the patient needs a medication, but for some reason this need is not recognized at the time of the patient-physician encounter and, as a result, no medication is prescribed at that time. Many studies conducted in Canada and beyond have also concluded that this scenario frequently occurs. For example, we know that many patients who suffer a heart attack (myocardial infarction) do not receive prescriptions for medications that we know can help to prevent a second heart attack.

The Prescribing Matrix[28]

		Prescription Indicated (Needed)	
		Yes	No
Prescription Written	Yes	Quadrant I	Quadrant II
	No	Quadrant III	Quadrant IV

What Is the Cost of These Problems?

Several studies have estimated the total economic impact of these problems related to medication use (or non-use). In 1995, two researchers in Arizona estimated the annual cost of these problems in the United States to be U.S.$76 billion.[29] Other researchers updated this study in 2001 and concluded that the costs had grown to U.S.$177 billion, more than double the estimate six years earlier.[30] Another study used similar methods to focus on costs in long-term care facilities (nursing homes). The total annual cost of adverse drug events in long-term care facilities in the United States was estimated to be U.S.$7.6 billion.[31] The authors of this study conclude that for every U.S. dollar spent on drugs in nursing facilities, U.S.$1.33 in health-care resources are consumed in the treatment of adverse drug events. Finally, in the only Canadian study to date, the cost of preventable adverse drug events in seniors was estimated to be approximately $11 billion annually.[32] So, overall, these problems do result in considerable financial cost to the health-care system, in addition to pain and suffering.

Which Medications Are Associated with the Most Problems?

By this point in the chapter, you may be wondering whether one or more of the medications you are taking is associated with adverse drug events. In essence, we can break down all adverse drug events into two general categories: problems associated with the medication itself (chemical properties) and problems associated with the use of the medication.

We often call the first type of problems *adverse drug reactions* or *side effects*. Generally, these are not preventable, except if, for example, it was known that a patient had an existing allergy to a medication and they received that medication anyway. As will be discussed elsewhere in this book, whenever you are prescribed a new medication, you should review these types of potential problems with your physician and pharmacist and ask for written information from your pharmacist. Each medication has its own side-effect profile and in some cases action can be taken to help minimize the potential impact of a side effect.

The second type of problems — those associated with the use of the medication — often are preventable. The Institute for Safe Medication Practice (ISMP) Canada has been tracking these preventable events, which they call *medication incidents*, in our country since 2000, reporting back to health professionals what they have found and working on strategies to reduce their occurrence. The following table contains ISMP Canada's list of the top ten medications involved in medication incidents that have resulted in death and/or harm. An important limitation of this data is that it is largely driven by the reporting of medication incidents in the inpatient setting, therefore it is not surprising to see drugs commonly given in the hospital setting in its list. It is also important to note that if you are taking one or more medications on this list, you should not stop taking your medication just because it appears on the list. You can always approach your physician or pharmacist if you have any questions or concerns about the medications that you have been prescribed.

Top Ten Medications Involved in Medication Incidents Resulting in Death and/or Harm in Canada*†[33]

Drug	No. of Incidents Resulting in Death or Harm	% of All Incidents Resulting in Death or Harm‡
1. Insulin	145	9.8
2. Morphine	133	8.9
3. Hydromorphone	115	7.7
4. Heparin	74	5.0
5. Fentanyl	55	3.7
6. Warfarin	51	3.4
7. Metoprolol	37	2.5
8. Furosemide	32	2.2
9. Potassium	29	2.0
10. Oxycodone	21	1.4

* Data from the Institute for Safe Medication Practices Canada database of medication incidents reported voluntarily by facilities and individual practitioners, for January 1, 2000, to June 30, 2008.

† A single incident may involve more than one medication.

‡ Percentages calculated on a denominator of 1,487, the total number of incidents resulting in death or harm.

Conclusion

In this chapter, we have presented evidence demonstrating problems with the health-care system and, more specifically, challenges with medication use. While there are many health professionals, researchers, and decision-makers involved in trying to improve patient safety in Canada and, fortunately, there have been some areas in which there has been a noticeable improvement, adverse events will always be an underlying concern in health care, given the nature of the risks involved. As we have reviewed, active personal involvement in care is one thing all Canadians can do, and it does help to reduce the risk of experiencing an adverse event. For those who are interested, we have also included several internet resources with additional information about these topics (see additional resources on page 16).

CHAPTER THREE

RUBBER-GLOVED
REQUIEM

The Canadian Health-Care System Gets a Checkup

A number of years ago, a five-year-old boy came to Dr. Rhonda's office to have stitches removed from a small laceration above his eyebrow. It was the commonest of childhood injuries: he'd collided with the corner of the family's coffee table a week earlier. As Dr. Rhonda worked, the boy's mother recounted their visit to the emergency department. She told of how each time one of the nursing staff entered the cubicle where they waited, the boy would whisper to his mother, "Is that the doctor?"

"No," she would say, "she's a nurse."

It was busy in the emergency department that evening, at least by 1990 standards. Finally, the physician, a salt-and-pepper-haired veteran, arrived. As he examined the laceration, his mother informed the boy that this was the doctor who would be stitching his cut.

"Mom," he said in a loud whisper, "that can't be the doctor. That's a *man!*"

In 1990, this story provoked laughs. At age five, Dr. Rhonda's patient could only recall ever having seen her as a physician and the notion of a male physician was foreign to him. But to many others, it seemed there were two types of health-care providers: doctors (men) and nurses (women). They were easy to pick out and everyone seemed to know what they were supposed to do. The doctor was a middle-aged man with greying hair, who wore either a navy blazer with gold buttons or a lab coat and wire-rimmed reading glasses that he peered over the top of as he rendered his (unquestioned) opinion. Nurses were women in white uniforms and starchy caps who took temperatures, passed out pills, and carried out doctors' orders. Things seemed tickety-boo: wait lists for health-care services were almost unheard of, as was the notion of a doctor closing his practice to new patients.

Fast forward twenty years and much has changed in the way health care is delivered in Canada. Female physicians have become the norm; there are at least as many women as men graduating from Canadian medical schools. The roles of many health-care providers, including nurses, have expanded considerably, and many new types of practitioners have appeared on the health-care scene. Today, a registered nurse might perform a Pap test, a procedure that once was done only by a physician. A pharmacist may, in some circumstances, prescribe medications. A physician's assistant may suture — or glue — a laceration like that of Dr. Rhonda's five-year-old patient, or a midwife might deliver his baby sister. A nurse practitioner could be the one to prescribe medication for his ear infection or monitor his grandmother's hypertension, and in the foreseeable future a nurse anesthetist may administer the general anesthetic for his dad's gallbladder surgery.

To the patient, particularly one accustomed to the traditional navy blazer and white uniform roles, it can be a bit bewildering. Not only might the registered nurse, the respiratory therapist, and the X-ray technologist at the local hospital sport the same uniform, but the gradual blurring and overlapping of the roles performed by health-care providers adds to the confusion for many health-care consumers.

That's where we come in.

In this chapter, the Canadian health-care system comes in for a checkup. We'll put on our rubber glove and poke and prod its nooks and crannies. Doctors know that making a diagnosis and deciding what needs to be done is highly dependent on taking a good history of the patient's current and past issues. We agree, and we'll crack open the Canadian health-care history books to help you better understand today's health-care landscape.

We'll look at the advent of new practitioners and the ways in which front-line care is evolving in many areas across the country. While we will offer fodder for revitalizing the system as a whole at the end of the book, at the conclusion of this chapter, we'll take off the glove and give you an eight-point prescription to help you better navigate the care you and your family need so you receive the safest and timeliest care possible.

Let's begin by asking why Canadian health care, once a shining national gem, now sometimes resembles a dollar-store ring?

The Canada Health Act

The Canada Health Act, adopted in 1984, sets out the rules of the road with which the provinces and territories must comply in order to receive federal transfer payments for the provision of health care to its residents. The rules require the provinces and territories to provide universal coverage for medically necessary physician and hospital services, without additional charges to the patient. The wording of the act, however, is as fuzzy as a forgotten fruit salad at the back of the fridge, and it does not describe how these services should be organized and delivered — that's left up to individual provinces and territories to figure out.

Universal, publicly funded access to physician and hospital services is, arguably, the thing that most defines the essence of Canadianism, even more so than beer commercial rants, Sidney Crosby, and short summers chockablock with roadwork and beaver-sized mosquitoes. In fact, several years ago, the CBC held a contest inviting Canadians to name the greatest Canadian who ever lived.

The winner was medicare founder Tommy Douglas. However, the premises on which the act was built back in the 1960s are now middle-aged and starting to creak and groan. Changes in the way health care is delivered since the act was adopted have meant gradual erosion in the proportion of services that fall under its umbrella, leaving Canadians with what is as far a cry from universal health care as Penticton is from Port-aux-Basques. In recent years, an increasing proportion of care is being provided in settings that do not fall under the Canada Health Act. The cost of physician and hospital services now represent just 41% of total health spending, compared to 57% at the time the act was adopted.

Many health-care services, therefore, are not picked up by the public purse, and their cost must be covered either by the individual using them or by a private insurance plan. Although some of these services may be at least partially publicly covered, many Canadians are responsible for costs associated with care in a long-term care facility, such as a nursing home, or provided in their home. Additionally dental care, eye examinations and corrective lenses, physiotherapy, chiropractic treatments, the use of crutches, or the provision of orthotics may be only partially publicly funded, or not funded at all.

And, of course, the elephant, or maybe that should be the bull-moose, in the room is prescription medications, which also are not covered by the Canada Health Act. Prescription drugs represent the fastest-growing item in health spending. More dollars are now spent on prescription medications than on physician services.

While every province has a pharmaceutical program to cover drug costs for its seniors and low-income residents, Quebec is the only province to require that its residents have either public or private drug insurance. Across the country, drug coverage is as uneven as a potholed road after a bad winter: a medication that is covered in one province or territory may not be covered at all in another and the processes by which new drugs are approved are unimaginably complex. Even for those with pharmaceutical insurance there is commonly a deductible: meaning that patients are responsible for the first several hundred dollars in drug costs each year before the insurance plan begins to pick up the tab.

Case Files: Seeing the Big Picture

At sixty-seven, Micheline felt that life had been good to her. She had retired from her job as a bookkeeper for a local auto parts dealer several years earlier, and she and her husband Bob, both in superb health, were looking forward to spending more time with their five young grandchildren. Micheline had always enjoyed quilting, and she planned to complete a full-sized quilt for each of their grandchildren over the next several years. She and Bob had never smoked, walked an hour each day, saw their doctor regularly, and often boasted that they were among the few people in their group of friends who were on no medications.

Micheline saw her doctor when quilting began to strain her eyes. At first she blamed poor lighting in their old farmhouse, but even with additional lighting, her ability to see fine detail continued to decline. Eventually she visited an ophthalmologist and explained that while she could see items at the periphery of her visual field, items in the centre were fuzzy and difficult to make out.

Micheline's doctor diagnosed macular degeneration, a deterioration of the specialized nerve cells in the macula, the portion of the "screen" at the back of the eye that allows us to see fine detail. Treatment was available, he told her, but the medication cost $2,000 per injection and she could need several injections to preserve her sight. Without the treatment, she would most certainly lose much of her vision.

Micheline and Bob were far from wealthy. They were making ends meet on their pensions, but there wasn't a lot left over. They were shocked to learn that the drug was not covered on their provincial seniors' drug plan; the private insurance that Micheline had while she was working was nullified when she had turned sixty-five.

"I thought I was paying taxes all those years so I would have health care when I needed it," she told friends, who hastily organized a dance at the local fire hall to raise money for the cost of the drug. They also put out collection jugs in businesses in the community. Fortunately, Micheline required only one injection of the medication, but the experience left her rattled and wondering what would become of their meager savings if she and Bob became ill in the future.

Catastrophic Drug Costs

Like Micheline in our case study, most Canadians assume that if they get sick, the costs of their care will be looked after. Sadly, it isn't until they face a life-changing diagnosis that many of us learn this isn't necessarily so. In September 2009, the Canadian Cancer Society released *Cancer Drug Access for Canadians*, a report that lays out the issue of catastrophic drug costs, a particular issue for Canadians dealing with cancer. It used to be that most drugs used to treat cancer were administered intravenously in a hospital. However, many newer drugs for cancer are taken by mouth, meaning the patient can take them at home. The cost of a course of treatment with one of these newer agents averages $65,000, and since they aren't administered in a hospital, where costs would be covered under the Canada Health Act, it falls to the patient or their insurer to pay for them. The report states that one in twelve Canadians face catastrophic drug costs — defined as greater than 3% of net household income. Even those with private insurance or government-subsidized drug plans face co-payments of as much as 20% of the cost of the drug — which can cost thousands of dollars a month. Clearly, while access to physicians and hospitals is supposed to be universal and covered, access to many other critical health-care services is not.

Universal Health Care: A Middle-Aged Muddle

Despite our universal health care, many Canadians are left in an impossible situation when faced with a serious illness. The system that was designed forty-odd years ago is just that — a system that was designed to meet our needs as a nation forty-odd years ago. Imagine the airline industry trying to land planes at Toronto's Pearson airport using a system designed more than forty years ago, or security personnel relying on practices and policies from the same era.

Today, new technologies, care options, and medications threaten to overwhelm both the public purse and the individuals who cannot afford to pay the costs of necessary services that are not covered. As public and private insurance plans attempt to control their costs, more and more of the costs of big-ticket drugs and other health-care services are passed on to patients. Patients in Canada, quite simply, are not covered for the wide array of health-care services they need.

Not that the provincial and territorial governments responsible for organizing, delivering, and paying for health care have an easy ride. In 1975, the provinces and territories spent, on average, slightly less than 30% of their total budgets on health care. By 2007, this had increased to 39%, with some jurisdictions expecting health spending to soon exceed 50%. There are even estimates that if total health-care spending continues to increase at its current rate, it could soon consume entire provincial budgets. A major wrench was thrown into the works when, beginning in 1996, the federal government began reducing transfer payments to the provinces. Despite a series of political gestures by the federal government, funding levels have never returned to pre-1996 levels.

While we spend a great deal on our health-care system, international data shows that the Canadian health-care system is not performing well and is not giving Canadians good value for their dollar. Our health-care system is the eighth wealthiest among twenty-eight industrialized Organization for Economic Co-operation and Development (OECD) nations, yet the Euro-Canada Health

Consumer Index ranked Canada thirtieth out of thirty in terms of value for money in 2008 and 2009.

So what has the fallout been of increasing health costs, reduced transfer payments to the provinces, and a health-care system that insures us for an ever-shrinking proportion of services? Not surprisingly, this has resulted in a number of barriers to access to care. We have already discussed some of the financial barriers to universal access. It is no surprise that in our vast nation, scarcity of resources tends to affect those living in remote areas the most. Even where resources seem plentiful, there may be issues with distribution. Nova Scotia, for example, has the highest number of physicians per capita in the country. However, their numbers are concentrated in the capital city of Halifax, which is the referral centre for many highly specialized services not available elsewhere in Atlantic Canada. Halifax is also home to the only medical school in the Maritimes (the first class of students at Dalhousie Medicine New Brunswick begins in September 2010), and many Halifax-based physicians are involved in teaching medical trainees, a task that reduces the hours they are available for direct patient care. Meanwhile, closures and service interruptions at emergency departments in more remote areas of the province are as common as fog off Peggys Cove.

Let's consider the stories of Lisa and James as we further explore issues of access to care.

Case Files: Desperately Seeking Doctors

Lisa, a mathematics professor in her early forties, called her family physician's office to make an appointment for her annual Pap test. She was upset to learn that her doctor, who had been there less than two years, had left the practice to pursue specialty training. Prior to that, the practice had been run by a male physician who left to do full-time walk-in clinic work. The physician before him also had had a short tenure before leaving to work in the United States. Lisa was very worried about missing her annual Pap test as she had had a history of cervical dysplasia — precancerous cells that, if caught early, are highly treatable.

Lisa was lucky. Eventually, her husband's physician agreed to take on Lisa and their three children.

Seventy-one-year-old James, a patient in the same practice, wasn't as fortunate. He'd had lymphoma several years earlier and was on a number of medications for high blood pressure, diabetes, and angina. After the doctor left without a replacement, he began calling various clinics in the city. None were taking new patients. The following month, his barber told him about a new physician in the area. James dropped by the doctor's office to ask to be added to the patient roster. After filling out a form listing his medical problems, family medical history, and medications, the office staff indicated that they would be in touch. After hearing nothing for almost two months, he called to inquire and was told that the practice was now full.

The next month, an ad appeared in the local newspaper indicating that another new physician was setting up a practice across the city. When James called, he was offered an appointment for a "meet and greet" interview. After outlining his medical history, the doctor told him he would not be able to take him on as he was trying to establish a practice with a balance between healthy individuals and people with complex or chronic disease. James, with his diabetes, history of high blood pressure, cancer, and heart disease, had been deemed too complex and time-consuming a patient.

Where Did All the Doctors Go?

Before the mid-1990s, except for some female family doctors who were in short supply, it was rare to hear of physicians not accepting new patients. Now few are, and Statistics Canada estimates that about 5 million Canadians don't have a family doctor to call their own. Among industrialized nations, Canada's doctor-to-patient ratio is one of the worst, at 2.2 per thousand, well below the average of 3. However, this wasn't always the case.

In August 1991, a report by Barer and Stoddart looked at the issue of physician supply at the request of governments who were concerned that the number of physicians was increasing more quickly than the general population and about the implications of this on health-care costs. In their report, Barer and Stoddart recommended a 10% reduction in medical school enrolment. This was quickly implemented.[34]

It was around the same time that the federal transfer payments to the provinces declined sharply. Reports of unemployed doctors were about as common as Haley's comet sightings in an Arctic blizzard. However, the government mantra became that there were too many doctors, and the excess number was driving up health-care costs. With the dual-pronged whammy of the perception of too many doctors and a sharp reduction in provincial health-care budgets, relationships between governments and physicians soured. Physicians' budgets were capped globally, meaning that provincial governments would only pay a set amount to the province's physicians as a group, regardless of whether additional patients needed care. Budgets were also capped individually, meaning that a physician could only earn a set income per year. After reaching their income cap, physicians would receive either no remuneration or reduced remuneration for the work they did for their patients the remainder of the year. Governments reneged on negotiated fee schedules with doctors, reduced their mobility by limiting billing numbers in areas they deemed to be "overserved" and brought in early retirement plans for senior physicians, a move that seemed sort of like chasing all the farmers away to keep people from overeating.

Not surprisingly, many physicians were outraged by what they perceived to be an anti-physician sentiment and at the prevailing attitude of government that physicians were "cost centres" rather than providers of valued services to people in need. Canada began bleeding huge numbers of its physicians to places that were delighted to receive them — particularly the United States. It is only in recent years that this net migration of Canadian-trained physicians to the United States has reversed itself. Since 2003, more Canadian doctors have returned to Canada from the United States than have left.

Around the same time as the reduction in medical school seats, physician training programs underwent a number of changes. Although historically a one-year internship after graduation from medical school had been sufficient to obtain a licence to work as a general practitioner, the requirement was increased to two years of post–M.D. training. Additional changes meant that medical students were required to choose their specialty much earlier in their training than in previous years. Traditionally, many newly trained physicians worked in family medicine for a few years, put in long hours caring for patients to consolidate their considerable education-related debt, and then returned for specialty training. However, these "re-entry" positions also declined considerably around the mid-1990s. Fewer students chose to enter family practice upon graduation, citing concerns about not being able to return later for specialty training, and contributing to the growing shortage of family doctors.

Around the same time, the numbers of women graduating from Canada's medical schools increased considerably. Although traditionally a male-dominated profession, by 1996, half of Canadian medical school graduates were female. Today at least half, if not more, of graduates are female. In the Dalhousie class of 2011, for example, fully three-quarters are women.

Female physicians work shorter hours than their male counterparts, and studies show that they spend more time with individual patients, leading some analysts to say that they are less productive than their male counterparts. A 2003 survey found that female family physicians work, on average, six fewer hours a week than their male counterparts. Among surgeons, however, the difference was only one hour a week.

It's no secret that medicine is a demanding profession. A 2003 survey carried out by the *Medical Post* and *Maclean's* found that 52% of family physicians indicated they would not choose the same career again. A Canadian Medical Association survey the same year found that nearly half of all physicians were in advanced stages of burnout; the numbers were worse for female physicians. Physician suicide rates are known to be double those of the general population, with the female physician rate quadruple those of others.

Not surprisingly, more recently trained physicians are looking at their burned-out older colleagues and saying, "Thanks, but no thanks" to the work habits that have landed them there. Newly minted physicians of both sexes are increasingly choosing to work shorter hours than their predecessors. In fact, it is estimated that these differences in work habits mean that it takes between 2.3 and 3 newly trained physicians to replace one retiring older one. While the Canadian Medical Association estimates that we need an immediate injection of 26,000 physicians to bring us up to the OECD average of 3 physicians per 1,000 population, if Canada were to adopt the policies of a number of European countries that limit the number of weekly hours a physician can work to forty-eight, we would have an additional shortfall of between 9,000 and 12,000 physicians.

One of the problems that may be contributing to the lack of family doctors taking on new patients is the way in which they are paid. Physicians have traditionally been paid using a fee-for-service model; they receive a set fee for a standard office visit regardless of the complexity of the patient's problem(s). This means that a physician receives the same fee regardless of whether their patient arrives for the visit with a simple earache or a long list of ailments. Moreover, an aging population with more chronic disease and advances in preventive health care — for example, monitoring cholesterol levels, a dizzying array of newly available immunizations, and increased understanding of the role of lifestyle factors — mean that many visits are longer in length than they once were. At one time, family physicians could count on a balance of longer, complex patient visits with quick, relatively straightforward ones. As overhead costs associated with running a practice — particularly in some large urban centres where office rent can be three times higher than in rural areas but where fee-for-service models mean doctors are paid the same amount — have escalated and physicians are less able to rely on a daily dose of quick-and-easy visits, the business model for providing a full-service family practice is in jeopardy.

This may, in part, explain the advent of walk-in clinics, and their focus on brief illnesses rather than complex disease management. Walk-in-clinic work, from a physician perspective, allows regular hours, no on-call, fewer managerial responsibilities, less unremuner-ated paperwork, and a robust income in comparison with the traditional family practice model. This is a particularly attractive option if you are a new grad with hundreds of thousands of dollars of debt and a young family. In recent years, there has been a migra-tion of many physicians who might otherwise be full-service family doctors toward episodic care such as that provided in walk-in clinics. No doubt, this has contributed to the current shortage of family doc-tors, and the trend is being watched closely. In 2008, for example, the British Columbia College of Physicians and Surgeons, the body that licenses, disciplines, and regulates that province's physicians, adopted a three-visit rule that stated that if a patient, particularly one without a family doctor, had three visits to a walk-in clinic, that clinic was required to assume responsibility for ongoing care of the patient, including follow-up of any chronic disease and investigations, and advising on and conducting preventive health manoeuvres.

One worrisome trend is what James, the "too complicated" sen-ior in our example above, experienced — commonly known as "cherry-picking." Many patients, and often those who are the most sick, report being repeatedly turned down by family physicians based on an initial interview or questionnaire. Provincial regulatory bod-ies have stepped into the fold in an effort to end this practice, which some say is a deliberate strategy for running a high-volume, high-billing practice by skimming off the patients who need shorter visits, leaving others — ironically, the people who may need them the most — in need. Although this does not appear to be a widespread prac-tice, it is clearly a concerning one. Physicians have been told in some areas that if they are accepting new patients they must, with a few exceptions, be open to "all comers" rather than just those likely to attend for minor illnesses.

Moving away from fee-for-service models and compensating physicians for the additional time required to care for complex patients is a step that is increasingly being adopted in agreements between physicians and governments. It is an attempt to ensure that patients with complex diseases receive the time-intensive care that is required by physicians looking after them.

Pandora's Inbox: Proliferation of Paper Imperils Physician Productivity

It seems a simple enough thing — you've been down and out with a nasty bug for a few days and thought it best to rest at home rather than make the people at work ill. But when you call your boss, she insists that you get a "sick note" from your doctor. You feel like asking if a note from your mommy would be okay since that's what you did in elementary school, but you manage to bite your lip. You know that the doctor doesn't have a cure for what ails you, but you sit in the waiting room, trying to keep your distance from the people that look a gazillion times worse off than you, all the while dutifully coughing into your sleeve because, heaven knows, these people clearly don't need what you have. And you're definitely not looking forward to having to pay the fee the doctor charges for the sick note.

Doctors across the country are beginning to push back against what they see as a proliferation of paperwork that does nothing to advance the medical well-being of their patients. Several years ago in Nova Scotia, it was estimated that if each of the province's 1,100 family physicians saw one patient a day for the purposes of providing a sick note, that translated into between twenty and forty full-time family physicians a year needed just to provide sick notes. In reality, there are many forms and other administrative duties that physicians do at the insistence of third parties that are not necessary for the medical care of the patient — sick notes are a mere drop in the bucket. See an opportunity to help ease the shortage of family physicians across the country? We do! Removing the requirement for sick notes from collective agreements between employers and their workers would help to recognize employees as the sensible adults they are and free up physicians to devote their time to those who are truly in need of medical attention, rather than forcing them to play truancy police.

Of course, beyond the challenges of finding and getting in to see a doctor, there are considerable barriers in access to diagnostic and therapeutic services. Given the fiscal restraints of governments, it is not surprising that it has been challenging to provide timely access to all advanced diagnostic and treatment services — such as surgery — to those who need them. Just as some Canadians must decide between the phone bill and paying for a prescription, governments are left to decide which services need increased funding, which might be able to hold the line, and which they may not be able to provide.

Lengthy wait times can unquestionably affect your overall health and quality of life. Many of us have, or have known of, an Uncle Bob who became almost housebound while waiting for a knee replacement or a co-worker who paid to have an MRI in a private clinic either here in Canada or in the United States when she developed multiple sclerosis–like symptoms and was told that her wait for an MRI in the Canadian public system would be measured in months, if not years.

While an OECD study of countries with wait times showed that physician availability is the most important factor in waiting times, the way hospitals are funded may be contributing to lengthy wait times for some services. Canadian hospitals have traditionally received block budgets that are population-based and relatively independent of how many of a particular service the hospital provides. Conceivably, a hospital doing ten lung transplant surgeries a year could be receiving the same budget as one doing ten times that number. Funding hospitals in this manner provides little incentive to providing increased volume of service. Under this funding model, it becomes financially disadvantageous for hospitals to do costly procedures.

There is little data on what has become a concern of many health-care providers in recent years — a perception of an increasing number of management staff at Canadian hospitals who perform no direct patient care, coupled with a declining number of hospital beds in what has been sometimes referred to as an increasing "desk-to-bed ratio." Not surprisingly, there have been calls for quantification of this phenomenon and a re-examination of the way in which hospital budgets are allocated by government. Linking hospital funding to the number of patients receiving a service is an idea that has surfaced in recent years, but clearly a system like this would need monitoring systems to be sure that hospitals do not cherry-pick patients who are less complex and therefore quicker to get in and out of hospital. Additionally, measures to ensure that providing increased numbers of services does not adversely impact the quality of care received would be needed.

Take a Seat, Please, the Doctor Won't Be Right with You

It has become difficult to open a newspaper in which there isn't a story about a patient who has waited too long for care. In 2005, the Supreme Court of Canada ruled that a patient could not be denied access to care paid for by private insurance when wait times for the public provision of this care were excessive. In its ruling in the case put forward by Quebec resident George Zeliotis and his physician, Dr. Jacques Chaoulli, who argued that the Quebec government should allow Zeliotis to pay privately to have hip replacement surgery since the wait in the public system was too long, the court said that "access to a waiting list is not access to health care." In the wake of this decision, many worried that the courts would open the door to the delivery of private U.S.–style health care. Since then, there has been some increased activity aimed at attempting to reduce wait times. In 2006, for example, the Quebec government introduced "care guarantees" for its residents for hip and knee replacement surgery, as well as cataract surgery. This means that if these services were not available within a defined amount of time, or "benchmark" in the public system, the Quebec government would pay for the surgery to be done at a private facility. Care guarantees have been used in a number of European countries in recent years and have resulted in marked reduction in wait times in the countries that have adopted them, and without exorbitant price tags. Denmark, for example, has a one-month care guarantee for elective services and a forty-eight-hour (yup, you don't need new glasses, we said forty-eight-*hour*) guarantee for cancer care. There has been some limited movement toward care guarantees in other Canadian jurisdictions. But they've been more like gestures or twitches than bona fide movement, as these have been only for a small number of services and the guarantees may include the cost of the care but often not the associated travel costs. As this book goes to press, the issue of care guarantees remains very much a patchwork across the country.

But beside the very human cost, what is the dollar cost of all that waiting? A study done by the Canadian Medical Association indicated that in Canada in 2007 the cost of waiting for care in just four areas — joint replacement, cataract surgery, heart bypass grafts, and MRIs — was $14.8 billion. This includes such costs as the patient's inability to work, medical appointments while waiting for definitive treatment, medication, services such as physiotherapy, and care by family members who may be forced to curtail their own work hours while caring for the patient.

Rebooting the Front Lines

In response to the barriers facing Canadians needing health care, a number of reforms have sprung up, particularly around the delivery of front-line health services such as those traditionally delivered by family physicians. In many areas, collaborative care teams have been established, with each member of the team providing a role in the care of the patient. Ontario, for example, has many Family Health Teams. Team members might include a nurse practitioner who can assess and diagnose many conditions, order investigations, and prescribe some medications. A registered nurse may conduct some health examinations such as Pap tests and well-baby visits, administer injections and immunizations, and provide counselling on lifestyle issues. A diabetes educator may provide counselling on diabetes management, and clinical psychologists could provide services to individuals with a wide variety of mental health issues. A team pharmacist may be available to provide advice on proper use of medications. Physician assistants, who perform a variety of roles, have been in use in the military and in Manitoba for many years, and there has been a resurgence of interest in adding them to the health-care team. Of course, patients are considered vital members of the team caring for them, a theme you will see us returning to again and again in this book.

Under these collaborative care models, as they are called, physicians focus on the management of illness, particularly complex illness. Often, physicians working in a collaborative care model are paid in ways other than traditional fee-for-service. This frees them up from the volume-oriented treadmill, which, as we have seen above, acts as a disincentive to providing care for complex and chronic illnesses. The jury is still out on whether these collaborative care practices are cost-effective and whether patient outcomes are improved over the long-term. However, these seem to be the wave of the future.

We Prescribe . . .

So what does all this mean for you, as a patient, seeking the best, safest, and speediest care for you and your loved ones? Here are tried-and-true tips to help you navigate the labyrinth that is the Canadian health-care system.

1. Be an active participant in your own health care.
We can't say this often or loudly enough: Ask questions and be sure you understand what you are being told. It is absolutely essential that you be a full partner with your caregivers. Know precisely what you have been told is wrong with you, the names and roles of all caregivers you are seeing, and the treatments — including medication names and dosages — you are receiving. Keep a written record and make sure at least one other person close to you is in the loop in the event you are too ill to answer questions. Don't assume that all the health-care providers you are seeing know all they need to know about you. Despite many advances in biotechnology, much of the health-care system still relies on an archaic system of paper record-keeping. Even where e-records are used, records in different care locales may not be integrated so they can "talk" to one another.

2. No news is not necessarily good news.
Moe, a thirty-two-year-old stay-at-home dad, saw his physician because of increasing fatigue. After chatting with the doctor, they both thought it likely that he was more tired than usual because of the stresses of caring for two young children and the financial and other strains that had arisen when Moe's wife unexpectedly became pregnant with their third child. However, they agreed that Moe would have a few blood tests conducted. When Moe didn't hear from the doctor, he assumed that his blood work had all come back and that the doctor had no concerns. Six months later, the doctor's secretary found a page containing Moe's blood work results behind a filing cabinet. It was the results of his thyroid function tests — indicating that Moe had an underfunctioning thyroid gland. After several months of treatment with thyroid replacement hormone, Moe was feeling much more like his old self.

No one, and no system for notifying you of abnormal results, is perfect. We suggest that whenever a test is ordered, you ask when the results will be available and book an appointment to go over them. Sometimes the lines between health-care provider roles can be a bit blurry, just as they can if you are seeing both a family physician and a specialist, or a physician and a nurse practitioner. In general, the responsibility for follow-up of test results lies with the person who ordered them, but sometimes one person may assume that another is communicating an abnormality to you. Always book a follow-up appointment with the person who has ordered your tests. If a follow-up appointment with a specialist isn't possible, say, because you live a long distance from their community, ask if you can follow-up with them by phone or with your family doctor, who should receive copies of everything that's been ordered and can act as a liaison with the specialist.

3. Chase their tails.

If you are being referred to a specialist or another care provider such as a physiotherapist, call a week or two after the decision has been made to be sure that the referral letter has been sent. In a busy practice, there is paper *everywhere*, with many forms to fill out, test results to order, and review and referral letters to write. Despite the best efforts of members of your health-care team, sometimes things fall off the radar. Or behind the filing cabinet.

4. Do your homework.

If you think the time you must wait for care is excessive, it's possible that the service you need is available elsewhere more quickly. Many provinces are beginning to post wait time information for various services on their department of health's website. Unfortunately, most physicians and their staff do not have the time or resources to fully research the shortest waits each time they are sending a referral and tend to refer to a small number of consultants and services they are familiar with. If you are concerned about the time you are waiting, do your homework and consider asking your physician if he or she will reroute your referral so you can be seen more quickly. You might also be able to determine from the provincial or territorial health department's website whether there is a care guarantee available for the service you need.

5. See the whites of their eyes.

While provincial Telehealth networks provide superb advice on a number of health-related matters, and can tell you whether you need to seek care, it is important that you always seek care in person if you are ill rather than asking your provider to prescribe over the phone based on your — or worse, your neighbour's — assessment of your condition. To further illustrate this point, let's look at the saga of Saul.

Saul was seen in his family doctor's office with a week-long history of a fever, weakness, and a cough. His doctor diagnosed a chest infection and started him on an antibiotic. Two days later, Saul's wife called to ask the doctor if she would phone in a prescription for something to help Saul sleep. "He put in a rough night last night," she said. "He was so restless. He needs proper rest to get better."

Judy, Saul's wife, wasn't at all happy when the physician insisted that Saul come in to be reassessed. "He's exhausted and weak. I don't know how I'm going to get him there."

Eventually, she acquiesced. Saul's physician thought he looked much worse than he had a few days before and she arranged for a few tests to be done. These showed a dangerously low blood oxygen level as a result of Saul's pneumonia. This was, doubtless, the cause of Saul's restlessness and inability to sleep. Saul spent almost a week in hospital — several days of which were in intensive care — before being well enough to go home. Taking a sedative medication at home would not only have masked the problem, it also could have worsened his pneumonia and, given his weakened state, increased his risk of an at-home fall.

6. Ask them to name names.

With the blurring of roles between health-care providers — and the similarities in uniforms — it is imperative that if you are receiving care in a collaborative care environment, such as one of Ontario's Family Health Teams or in a hospital setting, that you know clearly who each member of the team is and what their role is in your care. Likely, they will tell you, but if they don't, you absolutely must ask.

7. Choose your battles.

There are two points to make here. First, we know how very frustrating it is when you or someone you love is sick and worried and you have to wait for care. We believe you will get better care if you treat the people caring for you with respect. Dr. Rhonda recalls a situation a number of years ago in which the grandfather of an ill child raised his fist to her. (In case you're wondering, he did put it down before he used it.) Exhausted and worried, he lashed out at the nearest target — the physician who was trying to help his grandson. This may seem extreme, but patients and their families often take out their frustration on the very people who are trying to help, and sometimes in a very personal way. Clearly, this is not acceptable and making caregivers fearful of you won't result in you or your family member receiving better care.

Second, only ask for strings to be pulled when they really ought to be. Generally, priority for specialized services is given to those with the most urgent medical needs, with the specialist or the physician providing the service determining who is most in need. Sure, if your doctor calls and has a good reason for asking your care to be expedited, you might move up the line. If you believe your circumstances have changed, by all means you should speak up, but chances are everyone on the waiting list is as equally worried and unwell as you are. Best that you save your doctor's "trump card" for when you really need him or her to play it.

8. Ask for credentials.

Most health-care providers — such as physicians, registered nurses, nurse practitioners, and pharmacists — are licensed in the province in which they work. In order to obtain and maintain a licence, they must have appropriate training and must prove ongoing expertise and maintain appropriate professional standards in order to continue to hang their shingle. If the practitioner you are considering seeing is a non-traditional provider, we suggest factoring in whether the provider group is regulated into your decision.

9. Be a squeaky wheel.

Unless you've been vacationing on Pluto for the past decade and a half, you will know that the Canadian health-care system is in need of serious realignment in order for it to be able to meet the needs and challenges of the twenty-first century. Reforms to date have been insufficient to meet these needs, and sadly, changes at the political level are often driven by what might win votes. The next time there is a federal election, press the candidates who come to your door on the issue of federal transfer payments and the need for a national drug formulary and catastrophic drug coverage. Ask your provincial electoral candidates what they will be doing about the issue of care guarantees and the shortage of health-care workers. As a political issue, health waxes and wanes so make your candidates know that you will be supporting the party who delivers more than lip service on the issue of health reforms.

Your Medical Record: Who Owns It?

In a word, the record your physician or physicians keep in order to provide care to you is the property of the physician. However, you are entitled to see it unless — and this is a huge unless — in the judgment of the physician, what is contained there might be harmful to you. The physician must be able to prove in court what harm could come from allowing you access to your record. Your physician is obliged to provide you with copies of your record, or parts thereof, such as results of tests, with reasonable notice. However, this service is not insured under most provincial health plans and you therefore should expect to pay for the costs of generating the copies and any shipping costs. If you wish to view your record in person, your physician will likely request that a staff member be present while you do so. Physicians are required by law to keep records for ten years after you were last treated or, in the case of a child, ten years after they have reached the age of majority. After that time, the physician may destroy the file in a confidential manner.

Conclusion

The Canadian health-care system has evolved in recent years from one in which the traditional patient-physician-nurse roles have been replaced by multiple other groups of providers with blurred boundaries. Problems of access and excessive wait times are a symptom of a sick health-care system and one that is in need of rejigging in order to meet the needs of Canadians. However, armed with knowledge of your own health-care issues, a willingness to speak out and to shake bushes when they are in need of shaking, we believe you can receive very good care in Canada where and when you need it.

CHAPTER FOUR

FIRST,
DO NO HARM

Preparing for a Visit to Your Physician

One of the cornerstones of medical practice is the concept of *primum non nocere* — first, do no harm. This concept reminds physicians to always consider that any treatment offered to a patient has the potential to do harm and the risks and benefits of the treatment must always be carefully weighed against the risks of the patient's illness.

In the next few chapters, we will take an in-depth look at the interface between you, the patient, and your physician. First, our focus will be on arranging and preparing for your visit to your family physician's office — the most common entry point into Canada's health-care system. In this chapter, we will focus on how, when you are preparing for your visit with your physician, you can make decisions that will help you have the best possible health outcome.

We have said that a key component to safe and effective medication use is ensuring that medication is necessary and prescribed for the correct diagnosis. In Chapter 1, when we described a series of situations that led Paul to develop a near-fatal case of rhabdomyolysis, we introduced you to the concept of an adverse medical outcome as one akin to an alignment of Swiss cheese holes. In this chapter, we will discuss the role of the family physician and then walk you through the steps doctors take when they are making a diagnosis. We'll then turn our focus to the role of you as a patient working with your physician and his or her staff to reduce the chances of developing one of those Swiss cheese holes — an inaccurate diagnosis.

Since many errors can be prevented before you arrive in your doctor's examination room, we will offer suggestions regarding how to book and prepare for your visit with your physician. We'll challenge the convention that patients who get the best care are those who head to the doctor's office with a list of their concerns. We'll outline practical steps you can take to find a family doctor if you don't currently have one. Finally, we'll explore one example of a situation in which you just might be better off not seeing the doctor at all.

The Family Physician

For Canadians, a visit to the family doctor is the commonest point of entry into the health-care system. While the family doctor can solve many health problems, this physician also has several other critical roles. First, family physicians act as gatekeepers for access to other health-care services and providers. In Canada, for example, most specialists will only see patients on referral from another physician — often a family doctor. Although many other health-care providers such as physiotherapists, psychologists, podiatrists, chiropractors, and massage therapists can, and do, see patients without a physician's referral, many third-party insurance plans, such as those offered by employers, will provide coverage of these services only if a physician has initiated a referral.

Besides seeing you when you are ill, assisting with preventive health measures (such as screening for silent or early disease and providing immunizations) and referring you on to other health-care providers when necessary, the family physician has a critical role to play in maintaining your comprehensive health-care record. Family physicians maintain a record of illnesses and recommended treatments, and results of tests you may have had such as blood work or

X-rays. These would also include records of growth and development for children. If a patient is seen by a specialist, in an Emergency Department, or a walk-in clinic, a copy of the record of that visit as well as the results of any investigations, such as blood work or X-rays, should make their way to the family physician's chart. It follows that the family physician's chart should contain information on all prescribed medications.

If a patient has been admitted to hospital, the family doctor should also receive a summary outlining the details of the illness and its treatment, as well as a list of medications compiled at the time of discharge.

From Chief Complaint to Correct Diagnosis: How Your Doctor Gets There

In order to understand how to optimize your visit with your family doctor and increase the chances that your doctor will be able to make a timely and correct diagnosis, it is worth reviewing the process by which physicians make a diagnosis and arrive at a treatment plan that is then presented to you — the patient.

You arrive at the physician's office with a concern or a symptom. Physicians call this the *chief complaint*. For each chief complaint, there can be hundreds, if not thousands, of conditions or diagnoses possibly causing the symptoms. In medical school, physicians learn how to whittle away, through an organized process, at these possibilities to arrive at a single diagnosis or a short list of diagnostic possibilities known as the *differential diagnosis*.

After you describe the chief complaint, the physician asks further questions relevant to this complaint. This is known as *taking a history*. For example, if the chief complaint is a cough, the physician would likely ask about the duration of the cough and about the presence or absence of a fever or symptoms of an infection, such as a recent head cold. He or she might ask about the presence or absence of chest pain or shortness of breath and the characteristics of any sputum. If your doctor is not familiar with you, he or she might ask about smoking as well as general questions about your previous health history.

Many physicians consider history-taking to be the most critical aspect of their evaluation of a patient. A thorough history allows the physician to narrow his or her focus from a multitude of medical conditions that can cause a symptom, such as a cough, to a much smaller number. By the time the physician moves to the next part of the visit, the physical examination, most physicians will have narrowed the field to just a few diagnostic possibilities.

During the physical examination, the physician conducts an examination of relevant body systems based upon the information he or she has obtained during the history. This allows for further narrowing of the list of possible diagnoses. If the diagnosis seems clear, the physician may then suggest a plan of treatment. If the diagnosis is less clear, he or she may suggest investigations such as an X-ray or blood work to help arrive at a more firm diagnosis and treatment plan.

Using our example of a cough, let's look at two hypothetical patients and a doctor to see how this might unfold. Although both patients are ultimately diagnosed with pneumonia, the information that is gathered and the thought processes the physician uses to arrive at the diagnosis are different.

Amanda

Amanda is a twenty-three-year-old university student who comes to her family doctor's office over the Christmas holidays. Her chief complaint is a cough. She says that she developed a head cold about two weeks ago, just before exams, but now has developed a cough that is keeping her awake at night. Her physician, Dr. White, who has cared for since she was a child, knows that she is generally in excellent health and her only regular medication is the birth control pill. She has no allergies.

Taking Amanda's history, Dr. White learns that she had a fever for two days when her cold first began, and that it has returned in the last several days. She has no chest pain. She is mildly short of breath. She says that she is coughing up small amounts of green sputum and thought she saw a few flecks of blood in it on one occasion after she had been coughing particularly hard.

When Dr. White examines Amanda, she hears a few râles, which are snap-, crackle-, and pop-like noises at the base of Amanda's left lung. She briefly considers sending Amanda for a chest X-ray but decides she is confident that Amanda has pneumonia and needs treatment with an antibiotic. Although an X-ray would confirm this, it would not change her recommended treatment. She is otherwise in good health, and Dr. White knows that she will heed her advice to call if she is not improving over the next few days. Finally, she tells Amanda that it is possible the antibiotic she has prescribed could reduce the effectiveness of her birth control pill and she should use a backup method of contraception for the next several weeks.

Amanda returns to see Dr. White a week later, just before she is due to return to university. She tells her she is feeling much better. Her fever is gone and she has only a slight dry cough remaining. She is no longer coughing up sputum. When Dr. White examines her chest, she finds the râles have disappeared. Amanda returns to university and remains in good health for the remainder of the term.

Gerald

Gerald, fifty-seven, is also a regular patient of Dr. White. When he sees the doctor on the same December day as Amanda, he also has a chief complaint of a cough. Dr. White knows that despite a number of attempts to quit, Gerald has smoked up to a pack and a half of cigarettes each day throughout most of his adult life. He had a heart attack three years ago and is on a number of medications to reduce his risk of further heart problems but has difficulty affording the medications. He also has mild emphysema, a type of chronic obstructive lung disease.

From the patient history, Dr. White learns that Gerald has been waking up at night with sheet-drenching sweats. Like Amanda, he has a sputum-producing cough. Because of his lung disease, he has been coughing up white sputum most mornings for a number of years but over the past few months he has noticed that it contains increasing amounts of blood. Additionally, over the past week his sputum has changed from its usual white colour to green. He's been more short of breath and spent much of the past few nights sleeping in a chair as he found he was much less short of breath in this position. Dr. White also learns that Gerald has lost fifteen pounds over the fall despite a good appetite.

Gerald's chest sounds much different than Amanda's. It is difficult to hear his breath sounds — the usual flow of air in and out of the lungs — due to his chronic lung condition. There are also a few snap-crackle-pop râles at the base of Gerald's left lung, and Dr. White wonders whether she hears a few at the base of his right lung as well.

Although Dr. White was able to quickly diagnose pneumonia in Amanda, arriving at the correct diagnosis is more difficult in Gerald. By the end of their visit, Dr. White has a more broad differential diagnosis. Like Amanda, he could have pneumonia. But his history of heart disease means that he could have congestive heart failure, a serious condition in which the pumping action of the heart is diminished, causing fluid to back up into Gerald's lungs. He could have a flare-up of his chronic obstructive lung disease, which would require treatment with antibiotics and steroids. Even more worrisome is Gerald's weight loss and bloody sputum, which could indicate lung cancer.

Dr. White sends Gerald across town for a chest X-ray and blood work. By the end of the day, she obtains the results. Gerald has an elevated white blood cell count and an area of pneumonia on his chest X-ray. He also has a mass on his chest X-ray. Dr. White starts Gerald on an antibiotic and makes arrangements for him to have a CT scan to further evaluate his lung mass.

Medical Homes

Since millions of Canadians don't have a family doctor, we know we are making a big assumption when we are discussing your relationship with your family doctor. Later, we will discuss practical measures you can take if you have no family doctor, but we want to reinforce why you should have one — or make an effort to find one.

An emerging concept is that of the "medical home." This is defined as a regular physician or place of care (such as a healthcare team) in which the physician and staff are familiar with their regular patients and their medical histories. A medical home, by definition, can be contacted by phone during regular office hours and also helps to coordinate care received from other physicians or sources of care.

An international study conducted by the Commonwealth Fund concluded that individuals who have a medical home on average receive more positive care experiences.

Therefore, having a regular physician who knows your medical history, including your past and current medications, can help to ensure that your care is well coordinated and can help to reduce your risk of experiencing a medical error. Communication, both in person and by telephone, between physicians and their patients was also improved with the presence of a medical home. These findings suggest that having a regular physician can not only improve the health care you receive, but can also lead to a more trusting and personal relationship with those who provide care to you. Similarly, we strongly urge you to choose only one pharmacy to fill all your prescriptions. This allows you to build an ongoing, trusting relationship with your pharmacist. It also ensures that a complete, accurate, and up-to-date list of all your medications — and any possible interactions — is maintained.

Your Health Record: Paper Tiger or Digital Diva?

Most family physicians' offices in Canada still maintain traditional paper charts that are accessible only to the physician and other health-care providers in that particular clinic. Similarly, most hospitals and walk-in clinics maintain their own charts — most commonly paper as well. Pharmacies, however, mostly keep computerized records. At the present time, much of this information exists in isolation, with little ability for health-care providers to share critical medical data such as significant medical conditions, current medications, and allergies.

In contrast, Electronic Medical Records (EMRs) contain the same information in a digital format, with the potential to share necessary information between appropriate health-care providers in settings beyond the physician's office. This information is encoded in such a way that is highly secure — much more secure than traditional paper records.

These computerized health records offer advantages over paper charts. First, we're going to let you in on a poorly kept secret: physicians don't exactly have the world's greatest handwriting skills. Clearly, computerized records have a significant leg up when it comes to safety concerns related to legibility. And imagine never having to rummage through your wallet at the pharmacy for that folded-up square of hieroglyphics if your doctor could electronically submit your prescription.

Dr. Rhonda remembers very well a 2 a.m. drive to her office one frosty January morning after a patient of hers arrived in the Emergency Department with a suspected overdose. The patient was unconscious, the pharmacy was closed, and her office chart was the only source of information for Emergency Department staff regarding what medication, and in what amounts, her patient might have had at home.

Electronic records have additional safety advantages. For example, while it is virtually impossible for a physician who has paper charts to quickly determine which of her patients may be taking a medication that has been recalled by Health Canada or a drug manufacturer, a computerized record can quickly provide this information so the patient can be promptly contacted. Similarly, physicians' offices can quickly determine those patients who are due for important preventive procedures such as Pap tests and whether there are blood test results that have not returned as expected from the lab.

Established in 2001, Canada Health Infoway is an independent, not-for-profit organization whose mandate is to look at what is needed to bring the reality of EMRs to Canadians and their health-care providers. Infoway assesses what systems are working well and how these systems can be enhanced and expanded to expedite the development of EMRs. Infoway has set an ambitious goal of having, by 2010, an EMR for 50% of all Canadians that is available to the authorized professionals who provide their health care. Currently, only about 23% of all Canadians have any sort of electronic medical record. This is significantly behind New Zealand, the United Kingdom, and Australia at 98%, 89%, and 79%, respectively. Stay tuned . . .

As we have seen, the process by which physicians evaluate a symptom is much like whittling a piece of wood to a central core, which represents the correct diagnosis or a short list of possible diagnoses. In some situations, the characteristics of the patient — like Amanda — mean that the whittling process is very straightforward. In others — like Gerald — the process is more time-consuming and challenging.

The complexity of this decision-making process is not, however, solely dependent on an individual's previous health status. Some symptoms, by virtue of the huge array of diseases that can cause them, require a more complex decision-making process that has more potential for error.

Understanding this concept is key to knowing how to prepare for your visit with your physician and ultimately to you and your physician working together to arrive at a correct diagnosis and treatment plan.

To further illustrate this, let's acquaint you with two individuals: Aunt Minnie and Cousin Clem.

Aunt Minnie

Everyone has an Aunt Minnie. She may be your favourite aunt who always dresses in lavender from head to toe, plays Lawrence Welk eight-tracks from dusk to dawn, and wears pungent perfume that arrives at the family picnic about five minutes before Aunt Minnie herself. Or she might be a leopard-print aficionado, sipping Tequila sunrises at family weddings and leading everyone in the macarena. In any event, Aunt Minnie stands out. As soon as she walks into a room, everyone knows who she is. Even your long-lost cousin from Bora Bora who has only met her once can show up at a family reunion and immediately pick her out. She always looks the same, walks and talks the same, and acts the same.

It is believed the term *Aunt Minnie* was coined in the 1940s by a radiologist (a physician who is an X-ray specialist) at the University of Cincinnati. He used it to describe a medical case that had characteristics so clear and compelling there was only one possible diagnosis. In other words, if it looks like your Aunt Minnie, then it can be no one other than your Aunt Minnie.

Although this concept is one that is primarily used by radiologists, it provides a useful framework for understanding how all physicians make diagnoses. An illness or a medical condition that has features so unique that no other disease could possibly look the same could be called Aunt Minnie.

For example, impetigo, a common skin infection, would be an Aunt Minnie condition for most physicians. Impetigo commonly has a honey-coloured crust that is a dead giveaway to the trained eye. Shingles, a common painful skin rash caused by reactivation of the chicken pox virus that has been lying dormant in an individual's spinal cord, also causes a characteristic rash. The clear blisters on a red base appearing in a stripe along a nerve make this one another Aunt Minnie for most physicians.

Cousin Clem

Remember your cousin Clem? You may not. Clem is Aunt Minnie's son. Unlike Aunt Minnie, Clem prefers to fade into the background. He has mousy brown hair that is getting a little thin on top. He favours plaid shirts, khakis, and ball caps (to cover that bald spot). In fact, Clem is so nondescript that you're not certain you'd know him if you passed him on the street.

Many chief complaints that patients bring to their physicians' offices are much more like Cousin Clem than Aunt Minnie. Unlike the fiery red stripe of shingles or the honey-coloured crust of impetigo, chief complaints of fatigue, weakness, back pain, dizziness, or headaches are more like Clem. Even to the sharpest diagnostician, the causes of these symptoms are usually much less obvious. In doctor-speak, the differential diagnosis is much more broad. That means that for these problems, coming up with the correct diagnosis is much more challenging, time-consuming, and prone to error.

The Aunt Minnie–Cousin Clem Spectrum

Aunt Minnie
- skin problem
- sore throat
- earache
- fever
- eye problem
- suspected urinary tract infection — burning when voiding, voiding frequently
- lump

Cousin Clem
- fatigue
- stress or other emotional problems
- headaches
- back pain
- dizziness
- weakness
- chest pain

Booking an Appointment

Unless you are seeking care in a walk-in clinic or hospital emergency department most physicians' offices require that you book an appointment ahead of time. This means your first point of contact when you need to see a physician will usually be the receptionist.

Medical receptionists will commonly ask the reason you wish to see the doctor when you call to schedule an appointment so they can prepare for your visit. For example, if the clinic staff knows that you are coming to have stitches removed or to have a Pap test, they can have the supplies on hand that the doctor will need when he or she sees you. If you are coming in to discuss results of blood work, they can determine that the results have returned from the lab and are on your chart, ready for review. Additionally, knowing the reason for your visit helps to ensure that sufficient time is allotted for you.

As much as possible, whether you are booking a routine "well" appointment or a "sick" visit for a more pressing problem, try to book appointments with your regular physician. Unless your relationship with your family doctor is very new, he or she knows you, your background medical history, and the medications you are currently taking as well as any medication reactions or allergies you may have had in the past. Commonly, he or she will also be aware of the medical conditions of family members as well as how other facets of your life, such as the type of work you do or any recent emotional stress, might come to bear on your health.

In some clinics, doctors will pinch-hit for one another: if your own physician is unavailable, you may be offered an appointment with one of his or her colleagues. If your problem cannot wait until your own doctor is available, this is usually your next best option, as this physician should have access to your health record. Walk-in clinics are another alternative, but doctors there will not normally have access to your personal medical record — unless you are one of the lucky Canadians with an electronic health record.

When calling to book an appointment, be as forthright as possible about the reason you are coming in. You don't need to give the receptionist explicit details about your medical condition; a general idea should suffice. If you are being seen about a new problem or symptom, describe the symptom rather than telling the receptionist — and subsequently the physician — what you think is wrong or what you think the remedy is. For instance, Amanda or Gerald in the example above could simply say they have a cough, rather than they think they have pneumonia, or they are coming in because they need an antibiotic. Absolutely, when you see the doctor tell him or her that you have a cough, that you've had pneumonia on several occasions in the past, and that this illness seems similar, but allow the doctor to work through the usual history and physical. Even though this illness may feel exactly the same to you, there's a chance that it might not be pneumonia this time.

If the problem is of a very personal or emotional nature, just say so; that should be all the information the receptionist requires. Most receptionists will not push for further details.

Finally, it is important to realize that most receptionists do not have a medical or nursing background. While it may be tempting to ask them for medical advice, dispensing health advice is the role of the physician or office nurse, if your doctor works with one.

Talking the Talk: What to Say to the Receptionist When Booking an Appointment

Not so good: "I have a kidney infection and I need a prescription for an antibiotic."

Much better: "I have a pain in my side and a high fever. Could the doctor take a look at me?"

Not so good: "I am completely out of my pills. The little white ones."

Much better: "I'll be out of my blood pressure medication in a few weeks and would like to come in to have my blood pressure checked."

Not so good: "I just need to ask the doctor a quick question and get a prescription refilled." (Thinking, *I need to see her about my headaches, chest pain, the fact that I'm so tired all the time, a rash, and to have an insurance form filled out. Also, my husband is just about out of his little white pills and I'll get her to write the prescription while I'm in the room.*)

Much better: "I have a number of health issues that I need to see the doctor about. What do you suggest so that we have enough time to deal with them all? Also, my husband is running low on his diabetes medication and he needs to come in to have his diabetes reviewed."

Not so good: "I'm having terrible pain in my back. What do you think could be wrong?"

Much better: "I'd like to make an appointment to see the doctor about my back pain."

Rethinking "The List"

We have seen many magazine articles which suggest that you bring a list of your concerns when you visit your doctor. However, in our experience, one of the biggest challenges to working with your doctor to determine the correct diagnosis is having an overly crowded agenda when you see him or her. Most family practices book appointments of ten to fifteen minutes in duration. We'll explore reasons for this shortly.

In order to properly evaluate each symptom or problem a patient brings to a doctor, the physician must go through the process of taking a history, conducting an examination, considering whether additional diagnostic tests are needed, communicating the diagnosis or tentative diagnosis to the patient, developing and discussing a treatment plan with the patient including lifestyle or other non-drug treatments, and reviewing the need for, use of, expected effects, and potential side effects of any prescribed medications.

It is virtually impossible for a thorough assessment to be carried out for a lengthy list of problems in the course of a standard ten- to fifteen-minute office appointment. An overcrowded agenda sets the stage for any of the above steps to be short-changed, which could result in an inaccurate diagnosis and therefore an erroneous treatment plan. In "The Aunt Minnie–Cousin Clem Spectrum" we give a small sampling of a number of chief complaints commonly seen in family physicians' offices and show which ones are likely to be the more straightforward Aunt Minnies and which ones are more likely to be Clems. Problems that are closer to the Cousin Clem end of the spectrum are, from a physician's perspective, more challenging to thoroughly assess. We suggest that if one of these is your chief complaint you should plan to devote the entire allotted appointment time to working on this problem. Pick out the most troublesome one and let the doctor work through the whittling, which may include asking about other Clem symptoms. In our view, it's safest to focus on only one Cousin Clem problem or two Aunt Minnie problems and save the rest for another visit. Yes, your time is valuable, but your health is even more important.

Physicians prescribe medications for specific reasons and specific periods of time. If a medication is running low, the physician should reassess the condition for which he or she has prescribed the medication. The safest practice is to tell the receptionist that you are coming in for a review of your asthma or high blood pressure, for example, rather than for a prescription renewal. If you need a number of prescriptions refilled for chronic medical conditions — such as diabetes, heart disease, depression or other mental health issues, or chronic pain — plan to focus on just one of these conditions during your appointment, if possible.

If you have booked an appointment for yourself, remember the doctor has set this time aside for you alone. Occasionally, in the time that elapses between when the appointment is booked and the actual appointment, concerns may arise with other family members or loved ones. Your husband may be anxious to know the results of his hip X-ray or your granddaughter may have developed an earache. If additional family members who see the same doctor need attention, the best practice is to book a separate appointment for them so the physician has adequate time to deal with their medical concerns as well as yours. Rather than bringing them along to your appointment, give the office a call to discuss the best way to proceed. The doctor's schedule may permit you both to be seen. Avoid having an additional family member arrive unannounced; allowing the clinic to be prepared for both of you is the safest practice.

Finally, if you are planning to bring a number of concerns to the doctor, don't leave the most "Cousin Clem–ish" problem until the last. Besides being the toughest and most time-consuming to sort out, many of these problems can be the most serious. Hopefully, you have chosen to devote your entire appointment to this problem, but if not, bring it front and centre at the start of the appointment so that it receives the time and attention it deserves.

Why Is Ten or Fifteen Minutes All the Time the Doctor Has?

Family physicians are limited in the time that they have to spend with each patient largely because they are in such short supply. The Canadian health-care system is understaffed. According to the Canadian Medical Association, it would take an immediate injection of 26,000 physicians into this country to meet even the minimum standards set by the OECD. At the present time, it's estimated that approximately 4 million to 5 million Canadians don't have a family doctor at all. Since it takes the better part of a decade to train a family physician, it's not a problem that we can expect to be solved anytime soon. Those who are in practice typically have several thousand patients and a limited amount of time available to spend with each patient simply because the demands on their time are so high. A recent survey shows that Canadian physicians are increasingly frustrated with their inability to meet their patients' needs in a timely fashion and with their inability to provide care to those who don't have a family physician at all.

In our vision for the future, every Canadian will have a family physician. After many years of declining enrolments in Canadian medical schools, numbers have again begun to rise, meaning there is light at the end of this very long tunnel. But for now, the ten- to fifteen-minute appointment is the reality that most physicians and their patients must live and work within.

The One List You Should Never Be Without

While we don't advocate bringing a long list of ailments to your appointment, we do think you should always carry a list of medications you are currently taking as well as any allergies or reactions to medications you have had in the past. If you are visiting your regular family doctor, chances are he or she maintains such a list. However, since your medications may have changed if you have been seen by a specialist or admitted to hospital, the list might not be up to date. We suggest carrying this list with you at all times so it's readily available whenever you are seeing any health-care practitioner. An acceptable alternative is to bring all your medications in their original containers, or a list of all your current medications provided by your pharmacist. It is common for medications to be changed if you are hospitalized, and a follow-up visit with your family doctor after discharge from hospital to review the list of discharge medications the hospital provides you with is important.

"It's a Little White Pill, Doctor"

While physicians are well trained in the effects of medications, prescribing them, and monitoring their patients for side effects, many are not very knowledgeable about what pills look like. If Dr. Rhonda had a penny for every time a patient asked for a renewal on their "little white pill," she might not exactly be wealthy, but she would have an awful lot of pennies. She has had people bring in pills wrapped up in bits of tissue, or studded with bits of purse or pocket lint, necessitating a painstaking search through the pages of the *Compendium of Pharmaceuticals and Specialties* (*CPS*, or the "blue bible") in search of just the right "little white pill." We'll explore this in more detail in the next chapter, but it underscores the need for that medication list — and for knowing the names, appearances, and the reasons you are taking each of your medications.

Finding a Family Doctor

As mentioned earlier, if you have a regular family doctor you will likely have better overall health care as well as greater satisfaction with the care you receive. Ideally, all of us would have the opportunity to choose the family doctor who best suits our needs. However, few of us live in areas in which there is a surplus of family doctors.

Historically, many of us have "inherited" the family doctor who took over from our previous physician when he or she retired or moved on. However, it is becoming increasingly difficult for physicians to find replacements when they are closing their practices. In addition, it can be next to impossible to find a new physician after a move to a new community.

There is a glimmer of hope: In the 2007 National Physician

Survey, only 16% of family doctors indicated that their practices are completely closed; 20% indicated that their practice is completely open to new patients, and another 42% indicated that their practice is partially open, meaning they accept new patients under some circumstances.

If you find yourself without a family doctor, here are a few suggestions to assist you with your search:

- **Research.** Many provincial departments of health, colleges of physicians and surgeons (the bodies that license physicians), and local hospitals maintain lists of physicians accepting new patients. Call them or check out their websites. Be aware, however, that this information might not be up to date.
- **Don't go shopping.** You are probably in a better position if you don't have a family doctor than if you are looking to switch from a doctor you don't like. Some family doctors will not accept new patients who are looking to change doctors. Doctors like to avoid serial "doctor shoppers" who are chronically unhappy with any care they receive, but some will open their doors to patients who are new to the area or who do not have a family doctor.
- **Seek a physician with a special area of interest.** Some family doctors have areas of special interest or expertise and will continue to accept patients who allow them to use this expertise. For example, early in Dr. Rhonda's career her practice was closed to all new patients except prenatal patients. Sometimes she would also bend her own rules and accept patients who were planning to become pregnant in the near future.
- **Enlist your current doctor's assistance.** If your own doctor is leaving an existing group practice, chances are that you or your family may have been seen by one of his or her colleagues when your doctor was unavailable. In that situation, consider asking your doctor to approach his or her colleague on your behalf. In the small town where Dr. Rhonda works, several family

physicians who have recently left the community managed to "place" patients with significant medical problems with other physicians in the community by approaching them directly.

• **Ask another doctor.** If you don't have a family doctor, chances are you are receiving some medical care at a walk-in clinic or emergency department. Some physicians who staff walk-in clinics and emergency departments also have their own practices. Ask the physician seeing you if he or she does and would consider taking you on.

• **Use family connections.** Many family doctors will consider accepting family members of existing patients. For example, it is almost unheard of for a physician not to take on the newborn infant of a woman she cares for. Some will also agree to accept spouses or close family members of longstanding patients.

• **Network.** Do you know someone who knows a doctor? Maybe your next-door neighbour belongs to the same book club as a family doctor and would be willing to speak to her. Additionally, friends or family members who work in physicians' offices, hospitals, or other health-care settings may see family doctors routinely in their work day and may be willing to make a request on your behalf. If you are seeing a specialist physician, asking them to make a recommendation or advocate on behalf of the friend or family member is another possible avenue.

When the Best Remedy Is No Remedy at All

One of the most common afflictions for which North Americans seek medical attention is the common cold. A recent U.S. study indicated that upper respiratory infections, that is, the common cold, is the second most common diagnosis in family physicians' offices and the most frequent diagnosis in emergency departments.

We live in a society in which many of us have come to believe that there should be a pill for every ill. A head cold is a miserable nuisance, and in our fast-paced society we look for quick fixes even when there are none. When we feel miserable, it can be difficult to do the right thing — which may be nothing at all. This can be doubly difficult when someone we love, such as a child, is feeling miserable.

The common cold is caused by a variety of viruses, most often a member of the rhinovirus family. Adults average two to four colds a year, and young children may have upward of six to eight. Physicians are flooded with requests for antibiotics for colds. The reality is that antibiotics only kill bacteria and not viruses like those that cause the common cold.

Studies show that most over-the-counter remedies offer either limited benefit or no benefit at all. Additionally, they all potentially have side effects. Reports of serious adverse effects have prompted many agencies — such as Health Canada and the Canadian Paediatric Society[35] — to caution against using over-the-counter cough and cold remedies in young children. Additionally, reviews of a number of commonly used natural and herbal remedies failed to show any evidence of benefit from the use of these products.

A common cold usually begins with a sore throat, general aches and pains, and a low-grade fever. These symptoms resolve within a few days and are followed by nasal congestion, a runny nose, and cough within twenty-four to forty-eight hours after onset of the first symptoms. It is usually this second set of symptoms that prompt most patients to see a physician. Symptoms usually peak around day three or four and begin to resolve by day seven. Nasal discharge, appearing at the peak of illness, can become thick and green and may be easily misdiagnosed as a bacterial sinus infection that requires antibiotics.

Doctors often feel tremendously pressured to prescribe antibiotics to their patients for the common cold. A recent study showed the busier the physician, the more likely he or she is to inappropriately prescribe an antibiotic.[36] We suggest you think of a head cold as your body waving a white flag to tell you to slow down. Drink fluids, stay at home so you don't infect others, and wash your hands often so you reduce the chances of spreading the virus to your family and loved ones. Other than that, there's little — other than a tincture of time and lots of TLC for yourself or your loved one — that is guaranteed to work.

There absolutely are times when you should consult your doctor; many of these are outlined in "Symptoms You Shouldn't Ignore."

If you do see your doctor and he or she recommends an antibiotic, consider asking, "Do you think this would eventually go away without an antibiotic?" If the answer is yes, think about giving the antibiotic a pass for a few more days. The "just in case" antibiotic is probably not wise; a recent study showed that although antibiotics may be effective in preventing complications like pneumonia, 4,000 patients with the common cold must receive an antibiotic in order to prevent just one case of pneumonia.[37] And as we will see below, it just may not be worth the risk.

Hand It to Handwashing

The Public Health Agency of Canada endorses handwashing as easy to learn, cheap, and incredibly effective at stopping the spread of disease-causing germs. Handwashing is one of the pain-free ways to a healthier life. With fears not only of the common cold but also of pandemic flu, severe acute respiratory syndrome (SARS), and hospital-acquired infections abounding, it can feel like a possible outbreak is beyond your control. Yet experts say a simple way to reduce your risk is with good, frequent handwashing to prevent infectious diseases of all kinds.

Here's how to wash your hands properly:

- Wet your hands and apply liquid soap or clean bar soap.
- Rub your hands vigorously together, scrubbing all skin surfaces.
- Pay special attention to the areas around your nails and between your fingers.
- Continue scrubbing for at least twenty seconds.
- Rinse your hands and dry them well.

Symptoms You Shouldn't Ignore
There are, of course, times when you may need to see a physician since complications of the common cold can develop. See your physician if you have:

- a worsening earache
- shortness of breath
- swollen or tender neck glands
- chest pain
- a skin rash
- a worsening sore throat, especially with white or yellow spots on your tonsils or throat
- a cough that lasts more than a week or is causing choking or vomiting
- shaking chills or a temperature above 39°C lasting more than three days
- a headache lasting more than several days
- neck stiffness
- confusion
- blue lips, skin, or nail beds

Additionally, any child under the age of six months who has a fever or any child who is excessively sleepy should receive a medical assessment.

It's Just a Harmless Little Antibiotic, Isn't It?

While many of us think antibiotics are relatively innocuous drugs, they come with risks. While nuisance side effects like vaginal yeast infections and stomach upset such as nausea, vomiting, or diarrhea may occur, a much bigger problem is that of antibiotic resistance.

When an antibiotic is used to kill bacteria, it typically kills many but not all the bacteria. Through a process of mutation, those bacteria that are left behind have developed strategies to resist that antibiotic. As a result, they will be strong enough to resist that antibiotic in the future — either in that individual or in another person that the bacteria may be passed along to. This phenomenon is called *antibiotic resistance* and it's becoming a huge issue.

One such bacteria, methicillin-resistant *Staphylococcus aureus*, or MRSA, is becoming a significant problem in many of our hospitals and other health-care institutions.

Staphylococcus aureus is a common bacterium that many of us carry on our skin or in our nasal passages. Normally, it just sits there without making us sick. Occasionally, however, it can cause skin infections such as boils or impetigo. Antibiotic use is widespread in hospitals; after all, that's where individuals with the most serious infections usually receive care. As a result, a hospital-based strain of *Staph aureus* has emerged that is resistant to almost all antibiotics we normally use to eradicate it, even the heavy-duty ones. This strain of *Staph aureus* is called MRSA. While MRSA usually doesn't make healthy individuals ill, it can cause serious infections in frail hospitalized patients. Because of its antibiotic resistance, it's very difficult to treat.

In many hospitals, teams of infection control practitioners are now on staff to ensure that the very best practices and procedures are in place to appropriately screen for and treat individuals with MRSA and reduce the spread of MRSA within the hospital. According to the Canadian Patient Safety Institute, estimated costs for treating and isolating patients with MRSA infections were $82 million in 2004 and could reach $129 million by 2010. That's equivalent to the cost of approximately 12,000 hip prostheses for individuals in need of hip replacement surgery.

If that's not enough to make you think twice about dashing off to the walk-in clinic for an antibiotic prescription, consider another illness known as pseudomembranous colitis, which is caused by the bacterium *Clostridium difficile*.

Our large intestine contains a large amount of bacteria. These bacteria are of various types or "families" and many are important in keeping us healthy. Some, for example, produce vitamin K, which is essential in the formation of blood clots. Left to their own devices, these bacteria exist in relative harmony by keeping each other in check. A potentially harmful type of bacteria, for example, is kept from multiplying out of control by another type of bacteria. Think of it as a bacterial Mafia acting as bodyguards to keep any one type — or family — from becoming unruly.

Antibiotics can upset this delicate balance by killing off "bodyguard" bacteria. The unguarded bacteria may then rapidly multiply, and this in turn may lead to diarrhea. Usually our bodies look after this; balance is restored in time and the diarrhea disappears.

One of these bad-guy bacteria is named *Clostridium difficile*. Even his moniker sounds sinister. *C. diff*, as he's nicknamed, may quickly replicate himself if his bodyguards take a hit from an antibiotic. He has another trick up his sleeve, though; he can produce a toxin that makes the diarrheal illness even more miserable.

C. diff didn't used to be a big deal. While *C. diff* diarrhea made people feel miserable and a few became ill enough to require hospitalization, most people eventually got better either on their own or with the assistance of a *C. diff*–eradicating antibiotic.

A few years ago, though, *C. diff* turned nasty. Through the same process of mutation that leads to antibiotic resistance, *C. diff* developed not only antibiotic resistance, but also the ability to pass from one person to another — a characteristic this bacterium didn't have in the past. Additionally, the mutated bacteria developed the ability to make people much sicker than they previously had. In Quebec, for example, a mutated strain of *C. diff* was blamed directly or indirectly for more than 200 deaths in 10 hospitals in Montreal and Sherbrooke in the first six months of 2004. This mutated strain is still with us and continues to be a problem for hospitals in many parts of the country.

Conclusion

Evidence shows that having a regular family doctor is a key component of good health care. Making a correct and timely diagnosis in a family physician's office is dependent on teamwork between the physician and the patient. Clear communication with your family doctor's office staff and fostering a relationship with your doctor that allows him or her time to thoroughly assess medical concerns is essential. Bring just one or two concerns to your doctor's attention per visit, particularly if they are of a potentially serious nature or likely to require considerable time to sort out. Maintaining an up-to-date list of medications as well as any previous medication reactions and being knowledgeable about the medications you are taking are other important aspects of receiving the best possible medical care. Finally, be aware there are situations for which the best remedy may be no remedy at all.

CHAPTER FIVE

THE DEVIL IN
THE DETAILS

Navigating Your Visit to Your Physician

On the other side of the waiting room, a mother with three young boys in Spider-Man sweatshirts and scuffed sneakers looks up from a well-worn copy of a parenting magazine.

"Jacob," she says, "come, let me wipe your nose."

Jacob obliges and then wanders over to retrieve a toy from under the chair next to you. As he does, he lets loose a wet cough in your direction. He returns to his seat, tripping over the lacquered shoe of a man in a business suit who has been talking on his cellphone since he arrived ten minutes ago.

"Heavens," says the sixty-ish woman next to you, "the last thing I need is a cold. I'm just getting over double pneumonia. And I have to go in for a hysterectomy next month. Of course, that's minor. I had my bowel operated on last year. Cancer. The incision's been draining non-stop ever since. Bright green. Now I've got this funny pain in my head and queer dizzy spells. And my pee seems to have turned an odd colour."

She shifts in her seat. "What are you in for?" she asks, as though you're in a maximum-security penitentiary. Which is, in fact, how you're beginning to feel.

After twenty minutes in this mayhem, your brain is getting a little fuzzy. You try to think back to why you booked the appointment. Then your cellphone rings — your daughter has forgotten her math assignment and asks if you can drop it by the school. Returning your phone to your pocket, you glance at your watch and realize that you are going to be late getting back to work. You reach for your cell again to call a co-worker to ask them to cover for a few more minutes, but before you can you are ushered to a tiny, windowless room.

You begin to worry. Maybe you'll forget to tell the doctor some essential detail. Maybe he is going to find something seriously wrong.

After you finish with the doctor — who is not exactly renowned for his communication skills — you race back out to the waiting room for your coat so you can retrieve the math homework and get back to work. By the time you get to your daughter's school you realize you forgot to bring up the one thing you had wanted to mention to your doctor.

Sound familiar?

Help is on the way.

In this chapter, we look in detail at your visit with your physician. We discuss doctors' communication styles — commonly known as *bedside manner* — and give you practical pointers on how you can best work with your doctor if he or she is a little lacking in this department. We tell you what your doctor should know about you before he or she prescribes medication, review reasons medications are prescribed, and give you a checklist of what you should know about new medications before you leave the doctor's office. Finally, we discuss the booming business of complementary and alternative medicine and how to decide whether it is right for you.

The Medical Cast of Characters

At one time, if you didn't like your doctor's bedside manner, you found one who was a better fit. However, with the current physician shortage, that's not often an option. It would be great to have a doctor that looks like George Clooney or Uma Thurman, has the diagnostic skills of Dr. House and the genial manner of Dr. Marcus Welby, but they just don't exist.

In reality, many physicians are very good communicators but, like everyone, they may not be at their best all the time. Physicians do want to provide the best care possible and want you to understand what is wrong and what needs to be done to get you well. Sometimes, though, they need help and direction from you. We have created, for purposes of illustration, caricatures that show ways in which physician-patient communication can fail and how to get it back on track.

Dr. Halo Harrison

Dr. Harrison is a patient's dream come true. He is always on time. He spends a few minutes letting you voice your concerns before guiding you through the additional questions he needs to ask you. He explains your condition in clear and understandable language. When he prescribes medication, he makes sure you understand what it is, why you need to take it, how you can tell if it's working, what the side effects might be, and when you need to come back to see him. Before you leave he looks at you and asks, "Any other questions?"

Navigating a visit to Dr. Harrison

This doctor is (almost) too good to be true. Hang on to him.

Interrupting Patients

Early in their training, doctors learn the art of teasing out the "relevant" parts of what a patient has to say in order to obtain the information most useful to establish a diagnosis. Many patients, though, report feeling frustrated by doctors who interrupt them soon after they begin speaking. Investigators Beckman and Frankel showed that physicians interrupt their patients on average eighteen seconds after they begin to state the reason for their visit and that most patients do not complete their statements after being interrupted.[38]

So who is right?

Investigators in a Swiss clinic[39] asked physicians not to interrupt patients while they answered the question "What brings you to the clinic today?" The most common length of time patients took to finish speaking was fifty-nine seconds (patients who spoke longer brought the overall average up to ninety-two seconds). Overall, 77% of patients finished their initial statement within two minutes and only 2% spoke for more than five uninterrupted minutes. Physicians overwhelmingly reported that all the information patients gave during this time was relevant. The investigators concluded that physicians would be well advised if, at the beginning of interviews, they listened to patients without interrupting.

If your doctor is an interrupter, a quick "I'm almost done" or "Just give me a few more seconds to finish" might go a long way toward making sure your doctor hears your side of the story. Difficult as it might be to do this, it is important to both you and your physician that you are allowed to finish.

Dr. Jargon Jones

Dr. Jones looks you square in the eye when she delivers this diagnosis: "After a prolonged catarrhal phase, you now have a fulminant case of adenoviral pharyngitis complicated by profuse rhinorrhea. Nothing to worry about," she says, putting down her stethoscope. As she leaves the room, you reach for your cellphone to call your lawyer because you reckon you'd better get your will updated pronto.

What the doctor has actually said is that you have a viral sore throat and a runny nose.

Doctors spend so much of their time talking "medicalese" with each other and other health-care professionals they often don't realize that they are slipping into jargon when dealing with their patients. You, as a patient, deserve to be given information about your condition in clear language. You should never leave the doctor's examination room unless you have a complete understanding of what you have been told.

Navigating a visit to Dr. Jones
The first time Dr. Jones lapses into jargon, politely interrupt and say you don't understand. Ask her to explain in plain language. Don't wait until the end of the appointment.

It is perfectly acceptable — in fact, it's your right — to bring a family member or a friend to your appointment, as your advocate, if you think he or she might be able to help decode what the doctor has said if you're afraid to speak up.

Ask Dr. Jones to direct you to more information about your condition — such as a pamphlet or handout she has in the office or a reputable website.

If the doctor is a specialist, she is required to send a letter to your family doctor after she sees you, so booking a follow-up appointment with your family doctor to review this report is another option.

Immigrant Settlement Associations
Communicating with health-care professionals can be an even bigger challenge if you are new to a community, a culture, or a language.

Most urban centres in Canada have agencies that are contracted by Immigration Canada to provide a wide range of services to newcomers. The Metropolitan Immigrant Settlement Association (MISA), based in Halifax, for example, offers a variety of programs and services to newcomers to assist them in settling into their new culture or community. They offer English courses, programs to facilitate integration of newcomers into the Nova Scotia workforce, as well as services to assist individuals who are facing a serious illness or health crisis in their new community. Many hospitals have listings of physicians or staff members who know languages other than English and French, and provincial colleges of physicians and surgeons should be able to assist with finding a physician fluent in other languages.

Immigration Canada is a good starting place for learning about local available services.

A Word of Caution

When faced with a new and serious diagnosis, we commonly hear little except the diagnosis. A person who is told that they have cancer, for example, is unlikely to hear or understand much of what the doctor says after the word *cancer* or *malignant* has been spoken. In that circumstance, book a follow-up appointment to discuss questions that arise after you have had time to process the initial information.

Dr. Take-These-Pills-and-Don't-Ask-Questions Thompson

As doctors go, Dr. Thompson is a little "old school" in his approach. Although he may be of any age, Dr. Thompson has been slow to accept the notion that patients today want more information about their medical conditions and should be better informed as healthcare consumers. He passes you a prescription with illegible scrawl. "Here. Take these. Come back in three weeks." When you leave his office, you aren't sure whether he thinks your belly pain is from menstrual cramps, malaria, or a bad batch of mushroom marinara.

Navigating a visit to Dr. Thompson

Interrupt him with something like "I'm confused. Can you explain what's wrong with me and how this medication will help?" Using sentences that begin with "I" help to clearly establish what you need. For example:

"I'm not clear what the pills are for."

"I need you to back up for a minute so I understand."

Repeat questions such as these until you have all the necessary information.

As you would with Dr. Jargon Jones, if this doctor is a specialist, for further clarification you might also consider making a follow-up appointment to review the letter he sends back to your family doctor outlining his opinion and suggestions. Bring someone with you to the appointment, particularly if you have difficulties with your memory or become flustered talking to him.

Dr. Zachary Zoom

Dr. Zoom is a brilliant doctor who is very much in demand. He asks all the right questions, examines you, goes over his diagnosis and recommendations, but is in and out of the examination room so fast you thought you heard a sonic boom. By the time you remember that you had another question to ask, he's down the hall and in with the next patient.

Navigating a visit to Dr. Zoom

Preparing for a visit with Dr. Zoom is absolutely essential. If you have more than one concern you would like addressed, make sure you tell the receptionist when you call. When you see the doctor, tell him straight up: "I have two problems today." With this doctor, it is particularly important not to overwhelm the agenda, as outlined in the last chapter — bring no more than one Cousin Clem or two Aunt Minnie problems to the visit.

Some doctors' offices have a nurse on staff who may be a valuable source of information if you think of another question after the doctor has left the room. If the nurse can't provide an answer, he or she might be able to quickly interrupt the doctor or make arrangements to call you later.

Dr. What-Do-You-Think-Is-Wrong? Walker

You've just finished explaining your symptoms to Dr. Walker. She looks at you over the top of her glasses. "What do you think is wrong?" she asks. You're flabbergasted. If you knew, you wouldn't be here — you'd be, well, practising medicine down the street.

Dr. Walker isn't necessarily a lousy doctor. In fact, she very much wants to please her patients. In asking this question, she is most likely trying to allay your fears. In doctor-speak, patients often have a "hidden agenda" — something that is worrying them but they're afraid to say. For example, you may be tired all the time and more constipated than usual. You're really worried because this is how your mother was just before she was diagnosed with bowel cancer. What Dr. Walker is really asking is whether there is something in particular that you are worried might be wrong.

Navigating a visit to Dr. Walker
If there is nothing playing on your mind, just shrug and say, "I have no idea. I came to see what you think." If you are worried that your symptoms indicate a serious disease such as cancer, say so.

In summary, before moving on to discuss suggested treatments for what ails you with the doctor, you should have a good understanding of what she thinks is wrong. Asking questions as soon as something doesn't make sense, enlisting the help of friends, family, or the doctor's staff, and following up with a visit to the family doctor after seeing a specialist are all tried-and-true ways of being sure you receive all the information you need about what's wrong, regardless of the doctor's bedside manner.

Why Medications Are Prescribed

Let's now look at the reasons medications are prescribed and how you can be sure that both you and your doctor have all the information the two of you need to make an informed choice.

Most medications are prescribed for one (or more) of three reasons:

1. to treat or cure an illness,
2. to relieve unpleasant or uncomfortable symptoms, or
3. to prevent a future illness.

In the last chapter, we discussed the concept of *primum non nocere:* first, do no harm. When your doctor is making a decision as to whether a medication should be prescribed, he or she makes a judgment call based on the risks of the illness and the benefits and risks of the medication. In order to understand this balancing act, let's consider the three broad reasons medications are prescribed.

1. Treating or curing illness

Using antibiotics to treat pneumonia or chemotherapy to kill cancer cells are two examples of this. If your physician recommended an antibiotic to treat pneumonia or a course of chemotherapy to treat cancer, you likely wouldn't question the rationale for recommending that particular medication. Since both of these illnesses are potentially life threatening, it is acceptable that the medication has some possible side effects since the risks of these illnesses, left untreated, are so high.

2. Alleviating discomfort

Medications are also commonly used to relieve pain or other discomfort. Your doctor may prescribe medication, for example, to alleviate the pain of a sports injury, relieve indigestion, ease itching, or lessen anxiety. In many of these situations, your doctor may prescribe another medication to treat or to cure the illness and provide an additional medication to control unpleasant symptoms. Many of these symptoms or illnesses are what doctors call *self-limited.* This means that, in time, they would go away on their own. In this circumstance, the doctor needs to carefully consider the risks of the medication in relation to your discomfort.

When medication is being prescribed to alleviate discomfort rather than to cure a disease, you, as a patient, must be part of the decision-making process. It is always worth asking the doctor whether non-drug therapies such as lifestyle changes may be appropriate. It's also worth asking yourself how uncomfortable you really are. While it is absolutely appropriate to take medication to relieve discomfort if needed, the old physician adage that you may get 90% of your side effects getting rid of the last 10% of your problem is well worth considering. Consider Hal's story.

Hal, sixty-two, comes to the doctor with pain in both hips. An X-ray shows moderately severe osteoarthritis, the joint "wear and tear" that begins to rear its painful, ugly head in middle age. Although he has been slightly overweight all his life, Hal gained thirty pounds after becoming much less physically active when he retired from his job as a letter carrier last year. He knows he needs to exercise, but he hasn't been able to do so because his hips hurt so much. As a result, Hal's weight is continuing to climb. On occasion, he takes an over-the-counter pain medication, but it's not very effective. He'd been looking forward to retirement, but he feels miserable since the pain is now keeping him awake at night — and off the golf course.

Hal's doctor explains that while prescription medications are available to help relieve the pain of osteoarthritis, none cure or even slow the progress of the disease and it is essential to work to achieve a healthy body weight to reduce the stress on his arthritic hip joints. Down the road, surgery to replace his hip joints may be needed, but the wait can be considerable. After further discussion, Hal and his doctor decide he will attend a series of sessions with a physiotherapist aimed at both alleviating pain and developing an exercise program. He takes a brief course of pain-relieving anti-inflammatory medication but tries to use it only at night so he can rest and before his exercise sessions to alleviate exercise-induced pain. Over the course of nine months, Hal reaches a healthy body weight through a combination of diet and exercise. His pain diminishes to the point where he is able to manage it using occasional over-the-counter medications.

3. Preventing future illness

Increasingly, medications have come to play a role in the prevention of disease. While the old saying that an apple a day keeps the doctor away may well be true, an Aspirin a day taken under doctor's orders may keep the cardiologist at bay. The same holds true for a number of other medications and illnesses.

In some cases, your doctor is able to accurately determine that you are at increased risk for the development of illness. For example, doctors are able to look at age, family history, the existence of known heart disease or a previous stroke, high blood pressure, diabetes, cholesterol levels, and smoking history to determine your risk of a heart attack or stroke over the next ten years. In fact, you can do this as well — follow the links at www.heartandstroke.ca. Based on this risk, your doctor may — as part of a comprehensive plan that involves both non-drug and drug treatment — recommend medication to reduce this risk. Commonly, these medications work by lowering blood pressure or cholesterol to "target" levels known to carry a lower risk of future disease.

Another example is the use of medication for osteoporosis, a condition that causes thin, brittle, and fracture-susceptible bones. While many of us consider broken bones to be mere speed bumps in comparison to some bigger health problems such as cancer and heart attacks, the reality is they're actually major hurdles. As many as 50% of seniors with hip fractures die within the first year. Many others become so debilitated they cannot return to independent living and must enter a nursing home — not at all what most of us have in mind for our golden years. Bone density tests provide very accurate information on the risk of breaking a bone in the future. Both non-drug and drug therapies for treatment of osteoporosis, as well as programs to reduce the risk of falls, can make a difference. So does a healthy calcium-rich diet and regular exercise.

Using medication to reduce the risk of a future illness is one of the most significant medical advances of recent years. It's also the one that can be the toughest to accept: committing to taking a medication for a lengthy period of time — maybe even for life — when you feel perfectly well. With medication that is being taken to prevent future illness, it is vitally important that you have a clear understanding of why the medication is needed, that is, what the risks to you with or without the medication are and how monitoring or follow-up should take place in the future. Let's study Barb's example.

Barb, a computer programmer and lifelong smoker, was just thirty-nine when she had her first heart attack. Her father died of a heart attack in his forties. Barb was told she needed to quit smoking, and her doctor recommended a number of medications to reduce the risk of a future heart attack.

Although she initially took the prescribed medications, Barb worried about the possible side effects listed on the lengthy pharmacy printout. After conferring with several friends and checking the internet, she decided to forego the prescription and take an herbal medicine instead. She continued to experience chest tightness when she walked with her husband on the beach and suffered another heart attack when she was forty-two. Despite this, she continued to smoke, telling her doctor she could not stop smoking as it was the only thing that helped her to deal with the stresses of working and caring for her aging mother. She refused to change her stance on the recommended medications.

One summer morning, a co-worker found Barb dead at her desk, clutching her bottle of nitroglycerin spray.

What the Doctor Needs to Know About You to Safely Prescribe

Your mother was right when she told you that you should always wear clean underwear, wash your hands after handling money, and never, ever take another person's medicine. When your physician prescribes a medication, it is chosen and tailored especially for you. With more than 23,000 prescription drugs available in Canada, choosing the best medication for you is based on a number of factors. In the last chapter, we discussed the importance of an accurate diagnosis and your role as a patient in this. However, there are other pieces of information your doctor will need to know in order to make the best and safest medication choice. In some practices, a nurse or other staff member may collect this information from you on behalf of the doctor and the doctor may ask for further details as necessary.

Your family doctor is likely aware of your personal medical history, meaning that you will only need to review them with him or her if there has been a change. However, a specialist or emergency department or walk-in clinic physician probably is not. No matter how busy the doctor seems, make sure that he or she is aware of:

1. Chronic health conditions or previous serious illnesses
Let the doctor know about serious or chronic health conditions you have now or have had in the past. For example:

- Medication doses may need to be lowered if you are elderly or have kidney or liver disease.
- People with previous stomach or intestinal bleeding should avoid some medications commonly used to treat the pain of arthritis as they may reactivate the bleeding.

2. Names and doses of medications that you are currently taking, including any vitamins, over-the-counter, or complementary and alternative medicine (CAM)
In the last chapter we told you about the importance of carrying an up-to-date list of all medications you are taking. Rest assured we're not going to let you off the hook until you have one. Having this information readily available will reduce the chances of a reaction between a medication you are currently taking and what the doctor prescribes. For example, some complementary and alternative medicine (CAM) — which includes such things as herbal products and homeopathic medications — can increase the risk of bleeding if they are combined with prescription blood thinners used to prevent heart attacks and strokes.

The list should include the name of the medication, the dose (strength) of the pill, and how often you are taking it.

Medication Wallet Card*

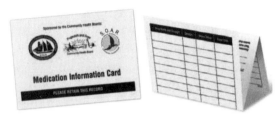

* This card is printed with the permission of Ann Keddy from the Cumberland Health Authority. It was produced in co-operation with the Pugwash and Area Community Health Board; Southampton, Parrsboro, Advocate and Region (SPAR) Community Health Board; and the Springhill, Oxford, Amherst and Region (SOAR) Community Health Board.

In Cumberland County, Nova Scotia, a local pharmacist and a family physician teamed up to develop a credit-card-sized medication identification card on which patients list their medications along with doses, how often they're taken, and when they were prescribed. There's also space to include any history of drug allergies, medical conditions, as well as names and contact numbers for next of kin, the family physician, and regular pharmacy. Simple and low-tech as this card is, information like this is absolutely invaluable to health-care providers.

Additionally, the doctor will likely want to avoid prescribing medication similar to one you are already taking. Many conditions, for example, are treated with a group of drugs known as anti-inflammatory agents. Among them are various types of arthritis, gout, sports injuries, kidney stones pain, and a number of gynecologic problems. If you are taking an anti-inflammatory medication for one of these conditions and develop a second condition for which this type of medication is commonly prescribed, it is unlikely that your doctor would want to expose you to the risks — primarily bleeding from the stomach — of taking two anti-inflammatory medications at once.

Be aware, however, that many physicians are not terribly know-ledgeable about the effects and side effects of CAM primarily because of the lack of credible information and good resources on many of these products. Your physician may not pick up on possible interactions between prescription medications and CAMS unless 1) you inform your physician about all the CAMS you are taking and 2) he or she is knowledgeable about these therapies or consults drug-interaction software. Otherwise, these interactions may not be picked up until you have reached the pharmacy.

3. Previous reactions to medications
As we'll explore in another chapter, not all reactions to medications are true allergies. However, it's worth making note of medications you've reacted to in the past, including what the reaction was. A good place to note this is on the medication list or card we suggested earlier.

4. Whether you are currently pregnant, breast-feeding, or planning to become pregnant in the near future
It goes without saying — but we're saying it anyway — that some medications can harm your unborn or breast-fed baby. Since many of a fetus's vital organs form before a woman may be aware that she is pregnant, it's important to mention if you are trying or planning to conceive.

Motherisk Program

The Motherisk Program at the Hospital for Sick Children in Toronto, created in 1985, conducts research and provides guidance to pregnant or breast-feeding women and their health-care providers regarding the safety or risk to the developing fetus or breast-fed infant, of maternal exposure to drugs, chemicals, diseases, radiation, and environmental agents. Visit www.motherisk.org as an excellent source of information or call 1-877-327-4636.

5. Financial issues that may make it difficult to afford medication
If money is an issue let the doctor know so he or she can factor this concern into the medication recommendation.

6. Any other issues that may make it difficult to take the medication as prescribed
Examples include a work schedule that would make it challenging to take medications on a regular schedule, significant memory problems that could cause missed medication doses, or difficulty swallowing pills.

Why Are Pills So Big?

Besides the medication, pills contain substances that hold everything together so they don't fall apart in the bottle as well as additives to make the taste acceptable. Additionally, "disintegrating agents" that help the pill dissolve in the stomach may increase the heft of the tablet. If you have a hard time swallowing pills, ask if a liquid form is available or if the pills can be cut.

Information, Information, Information: Don't Leave Without It

So you've met with the doctor. You've explained your symptoms and he or she has worked through a history and physical examination and come up with a diagnosis. Your doctor is recommending medication as part of your treatment. In order to safely take the medication, there are a number of things you should know or understand about the medication before you leave the office. Here is a checklist to guide you.

✔ What is the medication and why is it needed?

You should know the name of the drug as well as its purpose. For example, you should know the name of the antibiotic being prescribed and that it's being used to treat pneumonia, or the name of the medication the doctor has prescribed to lower your blood sugar to better control your diabetes.

✔ How, when, and for how long do I need to take the medication?

This can vary widely, even when medication is being used to treat seemingly similar problems such as infections. For example, you may need to take medication for a simple bladder infection only for a few days while you may need to take medication to treat a fungal infection in a toenail for many months. Some doctors mistakenly assume their patients know to take a medication for the long-term when they prescribe a medication to prevent a future illness. However, some patients stop taking medication their doctor intends for them to take long-term, such as blood pressure medication, when they run out of pills. This mismatch happens when the doctor and patient have both made assumptions — the doctor assumed the patient knew to continue to take the medication, and the patient assumed he was "cured" after the pill bottle was empty. It is important that you and your doctor are speaking the same language; be sure that when you leave the examination room you know whether the doctor intends for your medication to be taken short-term or long-term.

Your doctor may also give you information regarding the time of day you should take the pills and may also tell you about the timing of the medication in relation to meals or other medications. For example, some medications used to lower cholesterol are best taken with the largest meal of the day. Your pharmacist is also an excellent source of information about the timing of medication.

✔ Is any special monitoring needed while I am on this medication?
Most medications require monitoring to determine whether
they are working properly and safely. In some instances, a simple office appointment to confirm that your infection has
cleared or that your blood pressure is at target levels is sufficient. However, some medications require more invasive
monitoring. Many drugs commonly used to lower cholesterol,
for example, require blood work to confirm that your cholesterol has reached target levels and that it has not caused liver
irritation — a rare side effect of some of these medications.
Medications used to lower blood sugar in diabetics require
monitoring of blood sugar levels at home. Additionally, some
drugs require blood tests to determine that the amount of drug
in the body is appropriate, such as medications used to treat
epilepsy and some blood thinners. If drug levels are too low,
they won't work properly. If they are too high, there is a risk of
potentially serious side effects. People who live or work in very
remote areas or who have significant transportation challenges
may find it difficult to have the necessary monitoring. If that is
the case, ask your doctor to recommend another medication or
line of treatment.

✔ What are the possible side effects of this medication?
You may have noticed the CPS, the *Compendium of Pharmaceuticals and Specialties*, in your doctor's examination room. This
"blue bible" is the mainstay of reference books on medications
in Canada for physicians, pharmacists, and other health-care
providers. For each drug, there is an entry containing a myriad
of information on how the drug works as well as how it is to be
prescribed, used, and stored.

The process by which medication side effects are tracked and
reported means that a multitude of side effects make it to the
pages of the CPS. Many of them, though, are exceedingly rare
and some may have nothing whatsoever to do with a drug. For

example, somewhere in the CPS "reduction in sense of smell" may be listed. However, there can be many reasons why an individual's sense of smell may be reduced; sometimes this can occur simply as a result of aging. In another chapter we'll discuss the issue of medication side effects and how they are monitored and reported in Canada. However, it is worth knowing that many reported drug "reactions" that eventually make their way to the public, to health-care providers, or to the pages of the CPS may have nothing to do with the medication at all.

In recommending a medication for you, your doctor has weighed the risks and benefits of the medication against the risks of the illness and believes taking the medication is the best and safest option for you. What your doctor should tell you — or what you should ask — is what the common side effects are and whether there are any potentially dangerous or life-threatening ones you should be aware of.

It is important that you know what to do if you believe you are experiencing a medication side effect. Most times, you should not stop taking the medication until you have discussed it with your doctor. For example many women stop taking the birth control pill if they experience spotting between their periods. Stopping the pill in this circumstance is not only unnecessary, it greatly increases one of the risks of not taking the pill — an unexpected pregnancy! Your doctor, though, would likely want you to stop taking the pill if you think you have symptoms of a blood clot — a rare but potentially serious side effect of this medication. Ask your doctor whether there are any circumstances under which you should stop taking medication without checking with him or her.

✔ Do I need to come back to see you? If so, when?

In some circumstances, particularly if your illness is minor in nature, the physician may leave it to your discretion to return if the treatment doesn't seem to be working. In other circumstances, the doctor will want to see you to assess your response to medication and to monitor you for side effects. He or she will also want you to return if you feel your condition is worsening or not improving. Most doctors will also tell you to seek care if you develop "red flag" symptoms — he or she will outline these, if there are any — that could indicate a significant worsening of your condition or a serious medication reaction. For example, if you are seeing your physician for a skin infection, he or she may draw a line in ink around the edges of the infection and ask you to return if the redness spreads beyond the line.

If you are being seen by a specialist, ask whether you should follow up a newly prescribed medication with him or her or with your family doctor.

✔ Is this medication safe to take with my other medications?

Provided the doctor has an up-to-date list of your medications — including over-the-counter and complementary and alternative medication — he or she will make this determination before recommending a medication to you. While physicians generally have a very good working knowledge of what medications can safely be combined, some interactions may only be picked up if your physician or pharmacist uses drug interaction software, as discussed earlier in this chapter.

Prescription Refills

If your medication is running low, see your physician, who can then assess your response to it and monitor you for side effects. Together, the two of you can review the reasons you are taking the medication and decide whether you should continue taking it. In our view, this cannot be done over the telephone; a face-to-face encounter is needed to discuss how you are feeling, whether you are experiencing side effects, and to provide an opportunity for your physician to examine you. The best advice if you feel you need a renewal on a prescription is to make an appointment to see the doctor. It's also the easiest on the pocketbook since prescription renewals done without an appointment are not insured by provincial health plans, meaning that your physician will most likely charge for this service.

It is important to contact your doctor's office long before you are down to your last few pills to allow for the doctor's waiting time as well as the unexpected, such as winter storms, illnesses, or schedule changes.

If your own doctor is not available, ask whether a colleague in the same clinic would be able to see you. Walk-in clinics and emergency departments are also options, but the disadvantage — besides the long emergency department waiting times for non-emergent problems — is that staff members generally do not have access to your health record. Additionally, controlled substances such as narcotics are best prescribed by one physician only and many walk-in clinic and emergency department physicians will not refill these.

If you are on multiple medications and/or have a number of chronic health conditions, we strongly suggest booking a "medication review" appointment with your primary care physician at least once a year. Bring all your medications in their original containers, including any over-the-counter products you are taking. This review will help to prevent misunderstandings regarding discontinued medications and dosage changes, particularly if you are seeing a number of specialists in addition to your family doctor.

In some locations, and under some circumstances, your pharmacy may be able to issue enough medication to carry you through until your physician is available.

Complementary and Alternative Medicine

Complementary and alternative medicine (CAM) is an umbrella term for a wide array of health-care products, devices, and services that are not considered part of conventional medicine.

They fall under three general categories:

1. Products: Herbal and other remedies widely available over the counter at pharmacies and health-food stores. In Canada, these are regulated at the federal level under the term natural health products (NHPS).

2. Interventions: Treatments such as spinal manipulation and electromagnetic field therapy that are offered by a variety of providers, regulated or otherwise.

3. Practitioners: Various practitioners whose fields include naturopathy, traditional Chinese and Ayurvedic medicine, and many others. Many are unregulated, or regulated only in some provinces or territories, meaning that there may not be consistent policies regarding the training and certification needed to practise in these fields.

Here, we will be discussing only CAM products — referred to as natural health products (NHPS).

Over the past ten to fifteen years Canadians have embraced NHPS in much the same way as electronics aficionados have embraced Boxing Day sales. This has been fuelled in part by an increasingly informed public wishing to play a more active role in managing their own health, distrust and frustration with the mainstream health-care system, and a widely held perception that NHPS, being "natural," are therefore safe.

While many mainstream health-care practitioners accept and understand that people take NHPS for a variety of reasons, there is a great deal that isn't known or understood about these products. It's one thing to buy a computer printer at a Boxing Day sale based on a word-of-mouth recommendation or a colourful flyer; it's a far different matter to be putting a chemical into your body based on one.

It's important to consider that just because a product comes from a natural source doesn't mean it's necessarily safe. It also doesn't necessarily mean it's dangerous. Arsenic, for example, is a naturally occurring substance that none of us would ever dream of taking for its health benefits. And digoxin, a drug with many potential side effects that is sometimes used to treat heart failure, comes from the innocent-looking foxglove plant. The bottom line is that NHPs, like any medicines, need to be treated with respect. Anything that can create an effect within the body can also create a side effect.

Of course, NHPs are big business. Companies selling these products may make exaggerated claims on websites or glitzy infomercials in which an authority — often a celebrity or a "doctor" — provides a personal testimonial regarding the effectiveness of a product to treat a mind-boggling array of symptoms and illnesses. By and large, though, NHPs are not tested to the same degree as conventional medications in terms of their safety or effectiveness.

When mainstream medicines are being studied in anticipation of entering the Canadian market, the "gold standard" scientific study is the *randomized double blind placebo-controlled study*. It's a mouthful and it works like this: A group of individuals with a particular medical condition is divided into two smaller groups who are similar in important ways such as average age, number of males and females, and overall health. Half get the medication and half get placebo — essentially a "sugar pill." No individual knows whether he or she is getting medicine or placebo, and neither do the people who are conducting the study. That's the "double blind" part.

It's important to know that all medications have some degree of placebo effect. As many as 30% of people, in fact, will experience improvement in their symptoms or illness just from the act of taking a "medication."

Getting back to our scientific study, if 30 out of 1,000 people who received the placebo got better and also 30 out of 1,000 got better with taking the "real" medication, that drug would be determined to be "no better than placebo" and wouldn't stand a chance of making it onto pharmacy shelves. If, though, a significantly higher number got better on the medication than did on placebo, this would be considered pretty solid evidence that the medication works. Provided there were no serious side effects that outweighed the benefits of the drug, this drug might make it onto the market.

In Canada, whether a company marketing an NHP is required to produce randomized control trial evidence (RTC) of safety and effectiveness depends on what claims the company is making about the product. For most of these claims, the company is not required to produce evidence of quality RTC studies as is required of mainstream medications. Since 2004, regulations concerning NHPs in Canada have been tightened up considerably. However, in our view it is unlikely that most of these will ever be held to the same standard — proving safety and effectiveness with RTC — as conventional medications.

Some studies of NHPs have failed to show significant benefit. A recent review in the respected British medical journal *The Lancet* looked at a number of studies of homeopathic medicines and found that most of the time the effect of homeopathic medicines was no better than placebo.[40]

There can be other downsides to taking these products. Health Canada has issued warnings, advisories, and recalls about certain products, such as the use of eucalyptus in children and the potential for heavy metal contaminants such as lead in traditional medicines from India and Asia. Lead is "natural" for sure, but definitely not healthy. Other products have been linked to the development of serious illnesses and many can interfere with other medications. Equally worrisome is the fact that adhering solely to NHPs may result in delay of necessary, sometimes even lifesaving, treatment. We encourage caution and skepticism if a complementary therapy claims to treat or cure a disease for which mainstream medicine has no cure. Too often, we have seen patients spend extraordinary sums of money for unproven and ultimately ineffective treatments.

Consider Roscoe's story. Newborn Roscoe's parents were honest regarding their beliefs when it came to their family's health care — they preferred to use alternative medical therapies and would be seeking traditional medical care only when absolutely necessary. After a lively discussion about the roles of CAM and conventional medical treatment, the family received assurances from the doctor that he would be available whenever they sought his advice.

Several years later, Roscoe's Dad brought him to the doctor's office. Now a busy toddler, his parents were puzzled by a foul-smelling discharge from Roscoe's left nostril that had developed two and a half months earlier. A series of NHPs as well as restricting Roscoe's intake of dairy, wheat, and red meat had failed to clear up the problem.

After looking inside Roscoe's nose and a quick tug, the doctor removed a piece of a plush toy — most likely one that had fallen off a stuffed animal and been placed there by Roscoe. The discharge disappeared.

If you are considering taking an NHP, we suggest looking for credible information beyond that provided by the manufacturer or obtained by hearsay. The Complementary and Alternative Research Program of the University of Alberta, for example, conducts research and provides sound information on a number of products. Its website offers good information on the role of CAM in a number of common pediatric illnesses. For more information, visit www.care.ualberta.ca. Health Canada's website on NHPs also contains a great deal of helpful information, including claims made for these products, a list of licensed NHPs, and a list of single-ingredient monographs that describe the purpose of the product, the dose, and information on circumstances in which the product should not be taken.

Additionally, information provided by the manufacturer should include: instructions for use, information on side effects and interactions with other medications, and a list of situations in which the NHP should not be taken.

Unless this information is readily available for the product you are considering taking, it may be best to take a pass on it. And, again, if you are taking an NHP, be sure to let your doctor, pharmacist, and other members of your health-care team know.

Conclusion

So, you've successfully navigated your visit with your physician. You are confident that you've given your doctor the essential information that has allowed him or her to make an accurate diagnosis and prescribe a medication tailored to suit you. Although you may still not understand the hieroglyphics of the prescription in your hand, you understand what the medication is supposed to do, what side effects you might experience, how to tell if the medication is working, and what sort of follow-up you will need. Next up — a trip to the local pharmacy.

CHAPTER SIX

A PLACE WHERE EVERYBODY KNOWS YOUR NAME

Your Community Pharmacy

In this chapter, we will be reviewing one of the key places in most patients' health-care experience — the community (retail) pharmacy. More specifically, we will explore this unique health-care setting in more depth, including an explanation of what the pharmacist is actually doing behind the counter when each prescription is being filled. We will introduce some of the services that pharmacists are now offering across Canada and how these services may help you personally. We will provide practical advice throughout the chapter, including discussing previous research that has looked into why patients are, or are not, satisfied with their community pharmacy experience. And yes, we will also explain the title of this chapter.

Pharmacies, Pharmacies, Everywhere

It may seem as though there is a pharmacy on every corner. It is true that there has been a significant increase in the number of pharmacies in Canada in recent years. As of March 2009, there were 8,365 community (retail) pharmacies in Canada, an increase of about 1,000 since 2003.[41] Of all pharmacies in Canada, about 6 out of every

10 are chain and banner pharmacies such as Shoppers Drug Mart, London Drugs, and Lawtons Drugs. The remaining pharmacies are about evenly split between independently owned pharmacies and those found in grocery stores, large department stores, or big box stores such as Walmart, Costco, and Zellers. Community pharmacies tend to be both busy and profitable, although the profitability has decreased in recent years. The average pharmacy fills 60,000 prescriptions a year and has a net profit of $200,000.[42] However, at the time of writing this book, the Ontario provincial government has proposed legislation which would severely reduce financial compensation to community pharmacies in that province for generic drugs. If this legislation were to be enacted, it could dramatically alter the financial stability of pharmacies in that province.

As one might expect, one reason for this growth has been an increase in the volume of prescriptions dispensed by our country's pharmacists. We reviewed some trends in prescription drug use earlier, and these trends definitely have had an impact on community pharmacies. For example, in 2008, Canadian pharmacies dispensed 453 million prescriptions, or about 14 prescriptions for each Canadian on average.[43] As we will review later in this chapter, pharmacies are also offering more services than ever before.

So, is this increase in the number of community pharmacies good or bad? Pharmacists are well known as being the most accessible health professionals, and, indeed, there are many rural communities in Canada without a physician but with a pharmacist. If asked, most Canadians would likely say they would like to have both a physician and a pharmacy near their place of residence. However, while we have more pharmacies than ever before, we also have a shortage of pharmacists, similar to the situation we examined with physicians. In many cases, pharmacies are short-staffed and pharmacists work long hours; sometimes twelve-hour shifts without a break. According to one national survey, 49% of staff pharmacists and 50% of pharmacy owners and managers report a shortage of pharmacists in their own pharmacy.[44] So, we have a paradoxical situation where we have increased access to pharmacies in Canada and, at the same time, limited access to pharmacists themselves.

Another reason supporting the argument that an increase in the number of community pharmacies is a good thing for Canadians is that the community pharmacy is one of the three main entry points to the medication-use system for Canadians, as seen in the following table. The first entry point is self-selection, whereby a patient or

Summary of Entry Points to the Medication-Use System[45]

	Directed by	Medications accessed	Examples of access points	Severity of symptoms treated	Access	Safety concerns
Self selection	Patient or caregiver	OTC	Community pharmacy	Minor	Fast (within hours)	• Inappropriate drug selection • Incorrect dosing or application • Undetected interactions • Undiagnosed medical issue that might require other treatment • Lack of ADR monitoring
Prescribed use	Professional with prescriptive authority (i.e. physician nurse practitioner, dentist)	OTC and prescription medications (usually not IV or high-risk medications)	Physicians offices, walk-in clinics, ambulatory clinics	Minor to moderate	Delayed (e.g. wait time for physician office visit may be days to months) or fast (within hours) for walk-in clinics	• Worsening of condition or delay in treatment if there is a long wait time • Inconsistent monitoring and follow-up • Lack of long-term health data, incomplete medication profile and/or medical history, especially for patients who do not have a regular family physician • Time constraints in physicians offices and community pharmacies • Less opportunity for consultation
Managed use	Admitting physician (usually with multidisiplinary support)	Prescription medications, including IV and high-risk medications	Hospitals, long-term care facilities	Moderate to major	From intermediate to several years, depending on the urgency	• Miscommunication during patient transfers and between different groups of staff • Incomplete home medication profile or past medical history • Inconsistent or inadequate staff training • High patient volume • High-pressure, fast-paced work environment • Complexity of medical issues and use of high-risk medications • Inconsistent post-discharge monitoring and follow-up

OTC = over the counter, ADR = adverse drug reaction, IV = intravenous caregiver selects a non-prescription or over-the-counter medication for use. Most of this occurs in community pharmacies, and often the pharmacist is directly involved with the patient or caregiver in selecting a medication. These types of scenarios range from products for cough and colds, to foot care, home-care products, and diabetes monitoring supplies.

The second entry point is when the patient interacts with a health professional who can write a prescription (prescribing authority) and then the patient goes to a pharmacy to have the prescription filled. In the past, this has typically occurred through interactions with a physician or dentist. However, other types of health professionals are also gaining the authority to prescribe certain medications, although to be certain, most prescriptions are still, and will continue to be, written by physicians. There are differences among Canada's provinces and territories, but in some jurisdictions, midwives, nurse practitioners, extended practice nurses, optometrists, pharmacists, and podiatrists can prescribe certain medications.

The third entry point for access to medications is through an institution such as the emergency department of a hospital, the hospital ward, or the long-term care setting. Pharmacists are typically involved in the medication distribution process in all these settings, and often there is close interaction between the health professionals in these settings and community pharmacies. For instance, community pharmacies specially prepare medications in "bubble packs" for many residents of long-term care facilities in Canada. When a patient is admitted to a hospital, often a health professional in the hospital — a nurse, physician, or hospital pharmacist — will call the community pharmacy to get the complete medication record of the patient. And finally, when a patient is discharged from hospital, often he or she will stop off at a community pharmacy to have new prescriptions filled before heading home.

Which Type of Patient Are You?

Just as there are many types of pharmacies, from large "big box" pharmacies with a mini-grocery store and huge cosmetics section to small single-aisle pharmacies with just a few over-the-counter products, there are also different types of patients who go to pharmacies: Speedy Sue, Determined Dan, Chatty Ches, and Inquisitive Ida.

Speedy Sue
A Speedy Sue travels in and out of a pharmacy in a flash. She often has several children hanging off her (usually screaming) and wants to quickly pick up a prescription (birth control, perhaps?), pay for it, then dash back outside to her waiting minivan. She has no time for the pharmacist to tell her about her prescription and side effects to watch for. She may need one or two other things from the front of the pharmacy such as baby formula or postage stamps and may ask the pharmacist at the back of the store to ring in those items for her so she doesn't have to stand in line at a front cash register. If she does end up paying for these things at the front of the store, she may need to pick up some gum or candy to placate her children who are growing more restless by the minute. In her eyes, a successful trip to the pharmacy is to get in and out of the store in five minutes or less and for her children not to have broken anything.

Determined Dan
A Determined Dan may be in a rush like a Speedy Sue or more methodical. He comes into the pharmacy with one specific question in mind and will not leave the pharmacy until the pharmacist answers this question. He may have been sent to the pharmacy by his wife and, if so, he is going to make sure he has gathered enough information to answer any question he may be asked when he returns back home. His questions range from something simple, such as "What is the best treatment for athlete's foot?" to something more complex, such as "My son has these symptoms ... what do you recommend?" If he has time, Determined Dan will spend five, ten,

or fifteen minutes with the pharmacist, making sure he has reviewed all the alternatives for treatment and the costs, benefits, and side effects of all options. If he is in a rush, he may just purchase the first product the pharmacist recommends.

Chatty Ches

For a Chatty Ches, the pharmacy is the centre of the community, the meeting spot in town to see old friends. Time is not an issue for a Chatty Ches, as most Chatty Cheses are retired and would rather spend time in a pharmacy, looking at the new sale items, talking with the staff and old friends, rather than return to the drudgery of home life. A Chatty Ches not only knows all the staff behind the pharmacy counter by name, but also the names of all their children and grand-children, how the grandkids placed at the last dancing competition, and which products need to be restocked in the vitamins section of the pharmacy. After forty-five minutes in the pharmacy, Chatty Ches may buy a newspaper or nothing at all. He'll be back tomorrow, though.

Inquisitive Ida

An Inquisitive Ida often walks straight to the back of a pharmacy without looking around, asking to speak to the pharmacist directly. She often comes with a newspaper article, an advertisement from a magazine, or a printout from a website clenched in her hand. This piece of paper describes the promising results of a new drug or concerns about the long-term effects of an existing drug therapy. She asks the pharmacist if he or she has read this study and then asks a series of questions, such as "Should I stop taking my current drug and ask my doctor to start me on this one? Will my insurance plan pay for this drug? Do you know if this new drug has worked for any of your other customers?" Ida may follow up this visit with a telephone call later in the day or come back the following week with a new article about another drug.

What Is the Pharmacist Doing Behind There?

Have you ever wondered what the pharmacist and his or her staff are really doing behind the prescription counter? Sure, we know someone is counting pills and putting them into a prescription vial, but what else is going on? We will reveal this mystery by walking you step by step through the prescription filling process. The steps may vary somewhat among pharmacies but, in general, there are some key things that should happen with every prescription, regardless of where you take your prescription to be filled.

Let's start by describing the different individuals behind the prescription counter. First, there is the pharmacist. A pharmacist must legally oversee the prescription filling process and be physically present in the pharmacy, with the exception of some rules around remote dispensing (see "Prescriptions Without Pharmacists").

There are ten pharmacy schools in Canada and, in general, these bachelor of science in pharmacy programs are four years in length although students must have at least one year of university education before entering the pharmacy program. There is a general move in Canada in pharmacy education toward the doctor of pharmacy degree. Later in this chapter, we'll discuss the expanding role of pharmacists and describe the types of services that many pharmacists are now providing. Some pharmacists have taken over more of a management role and are also associates or owners.

Prescriptions Without Pharmacists

Ashlynn walks out of her family physician's office in northern British Columbia with a prescription for an antibiotic for an ear infection and heads down to the lobby of the large office building. Once there, she steps up to an ATM-like machine and places her prescription into the machine. She receives a prompt on the computer screen to insert her drug insurance card, which she does. Next, the face of a pharmacist appears on the computer screen. The pharmacist tells Ashlynn that her name is Kaylee and she proceeds to start a conversation with

Ashlynn, telling her about her new antibiotic and side effects to watch for. She asks Ashlynn if she has any questions about her new prescription. Even though Kaylee is physically sitting in front of a computer in Mississauga, Ontario, Ashlynn and Kaylee can easily see and hear each other. All the while, the prescription is being "filled" inside the machine as a label is being printed and attached to a prepackaged vial containing the right number of capsules of the right antibiotic. Finally, the prescription vial pops out of a chute in the machine. Ashlynn picks it up, retrieves her insurance card, and is on her way home.

Does this sound like a far-fetched idea for the distant future? It may, but PharmaTrust (www.pharmatrust.com) has this type of technology in Canada right now. In 2008, it conducted a pilot trial at Sunnybrook Hospital in Toronto, and the company plans on expanding this service in other locations. While it is unlikely we will see these types of machines pop up in every mall across Canada, they could be a very valuable alternative to a real pharmacy in certain settings such as remote northern communities.

Pharmacy technicians are key individuals in pharmacies as well. If pressed, many pharmacists will tell you that the difference between a good day and a bad day is the technician(s) with whom they are working. The educational level of technicians varies considerably, although recently a national examination has been developed for technicians so over time it is likely that passing this exam will be a requirement for all new technicians. The role of the pharmacy technician has also expanded in recent years with technicians now often performing duties that the pharmacist has performed in the past. Still, the pharmacy manager assumes responsibility for all actions of their pharmacy technicians and other staff.

Finally, some pharmacies may have pharmacy students working in the pharmacy completing the practical experience part of their university training.

The number and mix of the above individuals working in a pharmacy will often depend on the average number of prescriptions filled by the pharmacy. In pharmacies that do not fill many prescriptions daily (i.e., 100 or less), there may be a sole pharmacist behind the counter for the entire duration of the day. In very busy pharmacies (i.e., 500 or more daily prescriptions), there may be multiple pharmacists, technicians, and students working together simultaneously.

One other thing about the pharmacy you may have wondered about is why dispensaries are raised higher than the front-shop floor in many pharmacies. This originated at a time before security cameras to enable the pharmacy staff to more easily identify shoplifters. A secondary purpose was so that the pharmacist might more easily identify customers who may need advice in selecting an over-the-counter product. Many pharmacies still have raised dispensaries although most newly constructed pharmacies do not have this feature.

Moving onto the prescription filling process, when you take your prescription to a pharmacy, you will be greeted by someone at the pharmacy counter. This individual may be a pharmacist or pharmacy technician. This person will take a quick look at your prescription (or prescriptions, if you have more than one) to make sure the medication is in stock. Depending on whether this individual knows you, he or she will likely ask, at a minimum, if you have an insurance plan, your phone number, if you have any allergies, and, if the prescription is for a child, the age and weight of the child. He or she will also likely ask if you are planning on waiting for the prescription and, if so, will let you know how long it will take to be filled. While a majority of medications have already been manufactured by a drug company in a ready-to-dispense format such as a pill, capsule, tablet, or suspension, some medications must be specially prepared by the pharmacist and these typically take longer to be filled. These are called *compounds* by pharmacy staff. Often these are ointments and creams.

Next, the pharmacist or technician will look up your information (called the *prescription profile* or *patient profile*) on the computer and will type in the information from your new prescription. Most prescriptions in Canada are still handwritten by the physician in Latin abbreviations (e.g., bid = take twice daily, tid = take three times daily), although as we move to electronic health records, some physicians now print off a typed prescription from their office computer or even send the prescription electronically to the pharmacy. Pharmacists will likely tell you that trying to read the hieroglyphic-like handwriting on prescriptions is one of the more challenging aspects of their job.

It may surprise you that currently in most provinces in Canada, the pharmacist only has a record of the prescriptions that you have had previously filled at that particular pharmacy (the exceptions being British Columbia and Prince Edward Island). Moreover, even if you have your prescriptions filled in two different stores in the same chain (e.g., Shoppers Drug Mart), the pharmacist in one of those stores will not have access to the information from the other store. This is one reason why we strongly recommend that you have all your prescriptions filled at the same pharmacy.

Once your prescription information has been entered into the pharmacy's computer, it will communicate electronically with your drug insurer, if you have one. This is to ensure that the medication is included on your insurer's drug formulary (the list of medications your insurer at least partially pays for). As we reviewed in Chapter 2, drug formularies differ considerably from insurer to insurer. If the drug is not included on the formulary or requires special paperwork to be completed by your physician, the pharmacist will need to contact your physician before proceeding further. Even if the drug is included on your insurer's drug formulary, the pharmacist may receive other messages from the insurer that require his or her attention, such as a warning that the refill is too early to be filled. This, too, may require additional work for your pharmacist, such as having to phone your insurer to let them know that you are going on vacation and therefore it is okay that the prescription be refilled early.

At this time, one of the most important duties of the pharmacist occurs, even though it will not be evident to most patients. The pharmacist is using his or her education and experience to provide what is called *pharmaceutical care* (see "Pharmaceutical Care?") and will be looking for potential drug-related problems. The table on page 126 lists the eight types of drug-related problems and provides potential causes of each. For some of the drug-related problems, the pharmacist's computer software will assist, for example, by identifying drug-drug interactions or a dosage of a medication that may be too high. Other drug-related problems may be identified when the pharmacist interacts with you and asks you questions. As we reviewed in Chapter 2, unfortunately, drug-related problems are very common and can result in unnecessary emergency department visits and hospitalizations. The good news is that often these problems can be identified and resolved before you ever pick up your prescription. So, the pharmacist may have identified and resolved several drug-related problems with your prescription without you ever having been aware of this.

Pharmaceutical Care?

You've likely heard the phrase *medical care* used in conversations about health care. You've also likely heard the phrases *dental care* and *nursing care*. But *pharmaceutical care* may be a new term to you.

While the profession of pharmacy traces its roots back to ancient Greeks and Romans, it has undergone a significant transformation within the past twenty years with the introduction of *pharmaceutical care*. Since its introduction, pharmacists worldwide have embraced this concept, the training of pharmacy students has changed to reflect this concept, and pharmacists have changed their practice to provide pharmaceutical care.

What is pharmaceutical care? It has been defined as "the responsible provision of pharmacotherapy for the purpose of achieving definite outcomes that improve or maintain a patient's quality of life."[46] What this really means is that pharmacists are trying to move beyond simply providing a product (the filled prescription) and now try to provide a health-care service, working collaboratively with the other members of your health-care team to ensure that your medications are helping you to achieve the desired outcomes. This may seem like a simple enough process, but it can be quite complex and challenging if the pharmacist is to truly work alongside your physician to accomplish this.

So, the next time you see your pharmacist, ask to be provided with pharmaceutical care!

Major Types of Drug-Related Problems[47]

Category	Explanation	Potential Causes of the Drug-Related Problem
Untreated indication	Patient requires (has indication for) drug therapy but is not receiving it	• unrecognized condition • need for additional therapy • need for preventive therapy
Wrong drug	Patient has an indication for which the wrong drug is being taken	• wrong dosage form • drug that should never be used in the patient due to age, disease, and so on • ineffective drug • more effective drugs available • equally effective but lower-cost drug available
Suboptimal dose (dose too low)	Patient has a condition for which too little of the correct drug is being taken	• wrong dose (low) • frequency too low • duration too short • incorrect administration
Overdose (dose too high)	Patient has a condition for which too much of the correct drug is being taken	• wrong dose (high) • frequency too often • duration too long • incorrect administration

Adverse drug event/adverse drug reaction	Patient has a condition resulting from an adverse drug reaction or adverse event	• allergic reaction • incorrect storage • dosage increased too fast • adverse response to the medication that could not have been predicted • intolerance
Drug interaction	Patient has a condition resulting from a drug-related interaction	• drug + drug • drug + food • drug + laboratory tests • drug + herbs or drug-supplement • drug + alcohol • drug + smoking • drug + caffeine
Failure to receive drug	Patient has a condition that is the result of not receiving the prescribed drug	• drug not available • cannot afford drug • cannot administer drug (e.g., by swallowing) • cannot understand instructions • refuses to take drug
Unnecessary drug	Patient has a condition that is the result of taking a drug with no valid indication	• addiction or recreational drug use • non-medication therapy more appropriate • duplication in therapy • indication being treated no longer valid • treating avoidable adverse effects

During this time, the physical act of filling the prescription is underway. The pharmacy technician may print out the prescription label, retrieve the stock bottle containing the pills off the shelf, count the pills on a counting tray, fill the prescription vial, and attach the label and any auxiliary stickers, such as *take with food* or *may cause drowsiness*. Some busier pharmacies have automated parts of this process with automatic counting and/or labelling machines.

Once the prescription is filled, the pharmacist checks it against the original prescription written by the physician for accuracy. The pharmacist also double checks the unique number assigned to each drug product by Health Canada, the drug identification number (DIN). He or she assembles any written information about the drug product that he or she may wish to give to you, perhaps highlighting key points with a marker.

The final step of the prescription filling process is probably the most visibly apparent. This is where the patient or caregiver picks up the prescription, pays for it, and receives both verbal and written information from the pharmacist. "Things to Know and Do About Each of Your Prescriptions" could be used as a checklist with your pharmacist each time you pick up a prescription, to ensure that your pharmacist has discussed the key points of each medication you take.

Things to Know and Do About Each of Your Prescriptions

- DO know the name of the medication.
- DO know why you are using the medication.
- DO know what dose you are taking, when, and for how long.
- DO know what therapeutic benefit to expect and how soon to expect it.
- DO know what main side effects to watch for.
- DO know what *not* to take with the medication (e.g., other drugs, food, alcohol, herbal supplements).
- DO take the medication as directed.
- DO think of over-the-counter drugs and herbal supplements as medications.
- DO carry a complete, up-to-date medication list, including emergency contact information, at all times.
- DO talk to your physician, pharmacist, or another health-care professional if you notice undesirable symptoms after taking the medication or if you feel the condition being treated has not resolved or improved as expected.
- DO take a serious approach to medication. If you have any questions or concerns, ask your health-care professional.[48]

Of course, filling one prescription is not an isolated, stand-alone activity. Often the pharmacy staff will have several prescriptions in various stages being filled concurrently. Physicians may be calling in verbal prescriptions. Other physicians may be calling the pharmacist back in response to questions the pharmacist may have left with the physician's staff if he or she was not able to reach the physician. Other customers may want advice from the pharmacist on an over-the-counter product such as an herbal supplement. So, it is probably not surprising that filling a prescription typically takes longer than five or ten minutes.

The Evolving Role of the Pharmacist

In many ways, the profession of pharmacy is in a period of transition. As we have reviewed, the concept of pharmaceutical care has been widely adopted by the profession worldwide. As can be seen in the following table, both practising pharmacists and pharmacy students in Canada want to spend less time dispensing and working on third-party payer matters and on administration and spend more time in pharmaceutical care, talking with other health professionals, and conducting research. In fact, both pharmacists and pharmacy students would almost completely reverse the amount of time they spend on dispensing with the amount of time they spend on pharmaceutical care if they could.

The Real and Ideal World of Pharmacists and Pharmacy Students

Task	What Pharmacists Say They Do[49]	What Pharmacists Wish They Could Do[50]	What Pharmacy Students Expect To Do in Their First Job[51]	What Pharmacy Students Wish They Could Do in Their First Job[52]
Dispensing (filling prescriptions)	40%	23%	38%	17%
Direct patient care (counselling and pharmaceutical care)	25%	43%	19%	43%
Third-party payer drug plan matters	6%	0%	16%	5%
Administrative matters	4%	1%	12%	8%
Talking with other health professionals	6%	8%	10%	18%
Research	3%	7%	5%	9%
Other	4%	2%	0%	0%

Note: Numbers expressed as a percentage of total workday. Numbers do not necessarily add up to 100%.

It is not only pharmacists and pharmacy students who want to make these changes. Governments also want pharmacists to play a larger role in patient care. While Canada's provinces and territories are in various stages of implementing legislation that changes what pharmacists can legally do, overall there has been general consistency among the provinces that have already made these changes (New Brunswick, Alberta, British Columbia, for example). Other provinces such as Ontario are looking into similar changes. For some individuals, these changes are a long time coming, given the suggestions of Commissioner Roy Romanow of the Commission on the Future of Health Care in Canada, who said in 2002, "By truly integrating pharmacists into primary care, I believe we can improve the efficiency and effectiveness of drug therapy, reduce costs, and enhance patient care. The evidence is clear, the benefits are obvious and the time has come."[53]

While there are some exceptions, in general, physicians have been quite supportive of working more collaboratively with pharmacists. In 1996, the Canadian Medical Association and the Canadian Pharmaceutical Association (now the Canadian Pharmacists Association) jointly stated that the pharmacist has a responsibility to monitor drug therapy and to maintain records that document "progress toward treatment goals [if known]."[54] In 2002, the *American College of Physicians* and *American Society of Internal Medicine* released a position paper on the pharmacist's scope of practice and proposed an increased role for pharmacists, including having them serve as immunizers and participants in collaborative practice agreements with physicians.[55]

Finally, another factor driving change in the community pharmacy — and it may be the most important — is the evolving dynamic of how pharmacists are financially reimbursed for their services. Currently in Canada, third-party payers such as provincial drug plans and employer drug plans pay for most prescriptions. In 2008, public drug plans paid for 44.5% of all prescription costs, private insurers paid for 37.1%, while the out-of-pocket expenses of Canadians accounted for only 18.4% of expenses.[56] Over time, the percentage of all prescription expenses paid by third-party payers has increased, from 75.8% in 1988 to 81.6% in 2008. This is important, as over the past few years in particular, public payers are reimbursing pharmacists less for each prescription filled. This means that pharmacists are turning to other types of services to maintain financial viability.

Services Provided by Community Pharmacists

In this section, we will explore several different types of innovative services that many pharmacists are now providing in Canada. Because some of these services may be new to you, we will also briefly review some of the evidence that supports these services and how these services could benefit you personally. Certainly, not every pharmacy is providing each of these services, and, indeed, there are some pharmacies that are not providing any of these services. We will not be reviewing more traditional services offered by many pharmacies such as home prescription delivery and blood pressure clinics.

If one or more of these services interests you, we suggest that you ask your pharmacist whether the pharmacy provides these services and, if not, whether it is planning on offering these services in the near future. While some pharmacies may charge fees for some of these services, many are provided at no charge or your insurance company may pay for the services. It is really just a matter of finding out from your pharmacist which services are offered and how to access them. For example, how would you like to have a one-on-one thirty-minute session with your pharmacist to review each of your medications in depth? Provincial drug programs in Ontario and Nova Scotia now pay all or some of the costs of these sessions for certain people (e.g., seniors). Even if this service is not covered by your drug plan, your pharmacist may be willing to perform this service for low or no cost.

Callback programs

As the name suggests, a callback program is simply a telephone call from the pharmacist to you, typically three to five days after you start a new prescription. This service is almost always free (just ask!) and is a great way to have the pharmacist check on you to see if you have any questions about your medications that you may not have thought of at the busy pharmacy counter. The pharmacist will also check to see if you've developed any side effects from your medication and, if so, what to do about them. The pharmacist will call at a time that is convenient for you, and you can speak to the pharmacist from the privacy of your own home.

Studies that assessed the impact of these pharmacist callbacks have demonstrated that they are quite powerful. In 2006, one study found that pharmacist telephone follow-up improved adherence and reduced mortality by 41%.[57] Another study determined that a pharmacist callback program had a significant and positive effect on patient feedback, knowledge, medication beliefs, and perceptions of progress.[58]

Chronic disease management
Many Canadians have one or more chronic diseases, such as asthma, diabetes, or cardiovascular diseases. While these diseases are typically managed by a team of health professionals, often, in the past, the pharmacist did not have a real role to play, other than to fill prescriptions and provide some counselling. This has changed greatly in recent years with more and more pharmacists collaborating with other health professionals in chronic disease management. The services pharmacists provide in this area are quite wide-ranging, from helping patients with asthma use their inhalation devices and keep diaries, to doing in-store cholesterol checks and ongoing monitoring for patients with high cholesterol. If you have one or more chronic diseases, it would be worthwhile to ask your pharmacist if he or she provides any services or programs that could help you to better manage your condition.

One of the best known of these initiatives is the Ashville project in Ashville, North Carolina, which involved twelve pharmacy locations and several chronic disease states such as asthma, diabetes, and hypertension. Interventions with each of these disease states were made such that patients would receive education by a certified educator, regular long-term follow-up by pharmacists using scheduled consultations, and monitoring and collaborative drug therapy with physicians. Economic and clinical outcomes improved significantly for up to five years in the patients who were part of the programs.[59]

In Canada, the British Columbia Community Pharmacy Asthma Study involved thirty-three pharmacists trained and certified in asthma care providing enhanced care or usual care (control group) to patients with chronic asthma.[60] In the patients who completed the program, asthma symptom scores decreased by 50%, overall quality of life improved by 19%, knowledge of disease scores doubled, and emergency department visits decreased by 75%, as did medical visits. A patient satisfaction survey revealed that the study population was extremely pleased with their pharmacy services.

Collaborative primary health-care teams
This service — which is far more sweeping then the two services mentioned thus far — usually involves taking the pharmacist out of the community pharmacy altogether and having him or her work directly with physicians, nurses, and other health professionals in an office setting. Let us use a pharmacist — we'll call her Breagh — to illustrate this. Breagh works in a collaborative primary health-care team, spending her entire day investing one-on-one time with patients in a physician office or similar setting, without dispensing a single prescription. Pharmacists such as Breagh who are integrated into these physician practices are involved in chronic disease management, health promotion, and illness prevention, or patient self-management interventions, so as to optimize prescribing and use of medication.[61]

One of the largest studies to date of these types of practices was an assessment of the Integrating Family Medicine and Pharmacy to Advance Primary Care Therapeutics (IMPACT) project.[62] This study included seven Ontario group family medicine practices where pharmacists worked in conjunction with other health-care providers. Pharmacists had various roles within the practice sites, such that they would conduct individual patient assessments, including conducting medication histories; identify drug-related problems; develop, and monitor, care plans; and communicate the plan to the patient and interdisciplinary team. Upon request, these pharmacists also provided consultation to the family physician and other team members to assist in the individual care of patients, and provided educational presentations to team members and patients. Finally, these pharmacists also communicated with hospital and community pharmacists and other team members to ensure smooth transitions for medication-related care between care sites and recommended improvements to the medication-use system at the practice site. At least one drug-related problem was identified and assessed by the pharmacists in 909 (93.8%) patients. A total of 3,974 drug-related problems were identified, for an average of 4.4 drug-related problems per patient. The most common drug-related problems identified included patients in whom there were indications requiring a therapy but who were not receiving it (27.0%), patients who were not taking or receiving the prescribed drugs appropriately (16.5%), and patients who were receiving too low a dose of the drug (16.2%).

As you can imagine, this type of working relationship would be a pretty big change for most physicians and pharmacists in Canada. Successful collaborative primary health team care requires a shared understanding of roles and expertise for both physicians and pharmacists. Benefits to physicians of having pharmacists in a collaborative primary care practice include having colleagues to provide reliable drug information, group education, a liaison with community pharmacies, and an enhanced sense of team. In one study recently published in *Canadian Family Physician*, physicians' perspectives on collaborative practice twelve months after pharmacists were integrated into their family practices were positive overall.[63]

Health promotion and disease prevention
Pharmacists are the most accessible health-care professionals. As such, they are in a position to provide early detection of chronic diseases and to identify unhealthy lifestyles. They can help patients reduce risk factors by prevention counselling when appropriate (e.g., weight and diet management, exercise, and smoking). Pharmacists are a community-based knowledge resource who can help their patients understand the dangers of chronic disease and the importance of prevention. Pharmacists work with other members of the health-care team and can refer patients' chronic disease–related

issues to them. Furthermore, considering that treatment of chronic diseases often requires the long-term use of medicines, pharmacists are an invaluable asset in chronic disease management, as has been previously reviewed. The range of health promotion and disease prevention services offered by community pharmacies vary widely, from drop-in clinic days where seasonal flu shots may be offered, to screening for early signs of dementia, to ongoing monitoring and follow-up of drug therapy by the pharmacist.

The body of evidence in support of these types of activities has increased in recent years. A randomized control trial to determine the effect of community pharmacist intervention on cholesterol risk management in Western Canada was stopped early because of the overwhelming evidence showing the benefits of these services.[64] A review of community pharmacist effectiveness in smoking cessation interventions concluded that trained community pharmacists, providing a counselling and record-keeping support program for their customers, may have a positive effect on smoking cessation rates.[65] Another review concluded that community pharmacy–based services can help to reduce the factors that place patients at risk for heart disease.[66]

Immunizations

Pharmacists giving flu shots? Yes, but there are three levels of pharmacist participation in immunization services: educator, facilitator, and immunizer.[67] As educators, pharmacists regularly respond to specific questions about childhood immunizations, travel vaccines, and adult immunizations, as well as identify high-risk patients in need of specific immunizations. Pharmacists serve in this educator role today in pretty much all pharmacies in Canada. As facilitators, they assist in vaccine delivery through the traditional distribution of vaccines, as well as hold immunization clinics in the pharmacy. As immunizers, pharmacists provide immunizations to the public in those jurisdictions where this function is within the scope of pharmacy practice. In 2006, in the United States, immunization was being performed by pharmacists in forty-four out of fifty states.[68] At this time, however, pharmacists in Canada are just beginning to move into the role of facilitator and immunizer.

Patients seem to prefer receiving their flu shot from their local pharmacy where available. In a community pharmacy influenza immunization pilot, 80% to 90% of patients immunized reported that their pharmacy-based clinics were their preferred site for receiving immunizations. The most frequently cited reasons for this were convenience, less waiting time, not having to make an appointment, and easier parking.[69] Additionally, having the option to receive an influenza shot at a community pharmacy improves population immunization rates. In the United States from 1995 to 1999, influenza immunization rates increased by about 10% for states with pharmacists as immunizers compared to about 3% for states without pharmacists as immunizers.[70]

Medication adherence programs

Medication adherence can be defined as the extent to which patients follow the instructions they are given for prescribed treatments. Medications to treat chronic conditions typically require a degree of patient adherence to be clinically effective. Unfortunately, adherence with medications can be quite low, with reported rates ranging from 26% to 59%.[71] Furthermore, poor adherence can increase health-care costs, including avoidable hospitalizations.[72]

Many reasons exist for non-adherence to medication regimens, including (but not restricted to) problems with the regimen (such as adverse effects), poor instructions, poor provider–patient relationship (i.e., poor relationship of the patient to his or her physician or pharmacist), poor memory, low literacy level, and patients' disagreement with the need for treatment or inability to pay for it.[73]

What are the benefits of adhering to medication therapy? Patients who are knowledgeable about their medications, who are active participants in their own care, and who regularly ask questions can help prevent adverse drug events.

How can a pharmacist help with medication adherence? The methods vary and range from the simple to the complex. At the point of receiving your prescription, your pharmacist should explain the consequences of what may happen if you stop taking your medication and what to do if you develop side effects. If you find managing multiple medications frustrating, there are many different aids that pharmacies offer that you may find helpful. These include containers (dosettes) that have a different place to put your medications for each day of the week or even each time of the day you take medications. Many pharmacies will also prepare special "bubble" dosing of your medications where each dose of your medication is sealed in a foil bubble. If you find remembering to get your prescriptions refilled on time a challenge, many pharmacies now offer automated telephone refill reminders where you will receive a recorded message reminding you to have your prescription refilled. Finally, as will be discussed next, pharmacists can also work with you to see if there is a way to reduce the number of medications you are taking.

Medication reviews

Managing multiple medications is no easy task. It is easy to become confused when taking several (or many) different medications each day. Due to the different instructions and potential side effects and interactions, some Canadians may not be getting the most from their medications, may be at risk for potentially dangerous interactions, or may be taking medications they simply do not need. A *medication review* with a pharmacist or physician provides an opportunity for you to address any medication concerns you may have and ensures that you are taking only the medications you need when you are supposed to take them.

As of April 1, 2007, the province of Ontario began paying pharmacists for providing professional services in the form of medication review programs. MedsCheck provides an opportunity for patients (who are a beneficiary of the Ontario Drug Benefit Program [ODB] and currently taking three or more chronic prescription medications) to have a one-on-one thirty-minute consultation with their community pharmacist to help them better understand their medication therapy and to ensure that medications are being taken as prescribed. The service is free of charge to eligible patients, and pharmacies are compensated by the ODB.[74]

Similarly, in Nova Scotia, a Medication Review Service (MRS) was piloted in 2007 and launched province-wide in 2008. Eligibility requirements are similar; patients must be Nova Scotia Seniors' Pharmacare beneficiaries, taking four or more medications or one high-risk medication, and have at least one chronic disease. Pharmacists may submit the $150 MRS service fee once a year per patient to the NS Seniors' Pharmacare Program.[75]

Overall, medication reviews have been shown to significantly reduce the number of drugs used and the cost of therapy.[76] A 2000 randomized control trial determined that medication reviews resulted in changes to medication regimens in 47% of patients who had interventions (resulting in significant reduction in the number of medications per patient). Medication reviews also improved adherence to therapy in one study.[77]

Prescribing

The most controversial of the pharmacist services we are reviewing in this chapter is likely the emerging trend of pharmacist prescribing. Several provinces have granted pharmacists the authority to prescribe in some capacity, and in some countries, such as in the United Kingdom, pharmacist prescribing has become an accepted health-care practice. However, even where pharmacists have gained this authority, often there are tight limits and controls over what and when they can prescribe. Pharmacists certainly won't be replacing physicians as the main place Canadians go to get a prescription written!

One way to think of pharmacist prescribing is to look at this activity along a continuum. At one end, pharmacists prescribe over-the-counter and prescription drugs used to treat minor, self-diagnosed, or self-limiting conditions and provide emergency supplies of prescription medication. An example of this may be if you are taking a medication for a chronic condition, like angina, but have run out of the medication and you are unable to reach your physician (e.g., on the weekend). Your pharmacist has the authority to prescribe you a few pills to tide you over until you can see your physician.

At the other end of the continuum, some of the more advanced prescribing-related activities that some pharmacists can do under some conditions include monitoring and authorizing the refill of existing prescriptions; modifying prescriptions written by another prescriber to improve drug therapy (e.g., changing dose, formulation, regimen, or duration, as in dispensing a drug in liquid rather than pill form for a patient who has difficulty swallowing pills); prescribing medications for patients through delegated authority and collaborative practice agreements with a physician; and initiating or discontinuing a medication in collaboration with other health-care professionals providing comprehensive drug therapy management.

One potential advantage of pharmacists prescribing is to relieve the pressure on family physicians for patient visits related to refills and continuation of therapy for chronic disease. At the same time, regular, ongoing monitoring of your drug therapy by your physician(s) is critical. As displayed in the table on page 117, there are three primary access points to the medication-use system for patients. Currently, pharmacists are the primary contact for self-selection. As pharmacists move into prescriptive authority roles, they help to improve patient access to the second entry point — prescribed use. Still, some physicians are skeptical of the role of the pharmacist prescriber.[78] Arguments against pharmacist prescribing include having the same health-care professional both prescribing and dispensing represents an ethical conflict; prescribing requires an assessment that includes a proper history, physical exam, and ordering necessary diagnostic tests; and that prescribers must be prepared to treat any adverse effects from the prescribed medication. Overall, when surveyed, physicians are more comfortable with pharmacist prescribing when the pharmacist is known to them (has a well-established relationship).[79] This certainly follows what we are arguing for throughout this book — the need for seamless, collaborative practice between all health professionals. As we have suggested, physicians will, and should, remain the primary prescribers in Canada.

How to Increase Your Satisfaction with Your Pharmacy

Now that we have reviewed what goes on in a pharmacy and some of the novel services pharmacies are providing in Canada, let's turn to the topic of satisfaction with pharmacies. Over the past fifteen years or so, a lot of research has attempted to answer the question "What causes a patient to be highly satisfied with a pharmacy?" Our goal in including this topic is to increase the likelihood that you will be highly satisfied with your pharmacy experience and in better health as a result. We also realize that some of you reading this may not be in a position to choose your pharmacy. Perhaps there is only one pharmacy in your community or within reasonable distance to your home. You may be choosing your pharmacy solely based on convenience, whether it is due to location or hours of operation. For others, you may already be very satisfied with your pharmacist and pharmacy and have no desire to switch. However, we know there will be some readers who will be interested in optimizing their experience with their pharmacy. Regardless of which of the above sentences best describes you, we encourage you to read this section to get the most out of your community pharmacy experience.

Satisfaction versus expectations
One way to think about satisfaction is *the disconfirmation of expectations*; that is, we are satisfied when our expectations are exceeded and are dissatisfied when our expectations are not met. For example, you are likely to be satisfied with an experience at a restaurant

during an evening out when the level of service provided and the quality of the food exceeds your expectations. In the health-care context, you are likely to be satisfied at a pharmacy if the service was prompt, the pharmacist was courteous, and all your questions were answered satisfactorily. Admittedly, the parallels between satisfaction in health care and other industries may not be perfect since health care is not a typical commodity, such as purchasing a meal at a restaurant. Still, researchers doing work in this area tell us there are important lessons to learn from studying satisfaction in health care.

Why satisfaction in health care is so important

At this point you may be saying to yourself, "Okay, yes, I'd like to be highly satisfied with my health-care experiences, but how do I achieve it?" What is interesting about the concept of satisfaction is that many health-care researchers have shown how satisfaction relates to many other things in health care, including patient outcomes.

In their review of the patient satisfaction literature, two researchers observed that satisfied patients are more likely to continue using health-care services, maintain a relationship with a specific health-care provider (such as a physician, pharmacist, or dentist), adhere to their medical regimens (including medications), participate in their own treatment, and co-operate with their health-care providers. They conclude that "while research has not yet found a simple, direct correlation between patient satisfaction and improved outcome, satisfied patients seem more likely to comply with their treatment. Levels of patient satisfaction and patient compliance are presumed to subsequently affect other outcomes, such as the patient's health status, continuity of care, and the frequency and length of hospitalization."[80] So, it is clear that satisfaction in health care is a serious topic with important implications.

What causes patients to be satisfied with pharmacies?

Given that patient satisfaction is such an important concept in health care, let's take a closer look at the community pharmacy setting and see which factors influence whether a patient is, or is not, satisfied. Fortunately, in recent years, there has been considerable research studying the factors that influence the satisfaction of patients with their pharmacy experience.[81] We will now summarize this research for you.

First, access seems critical. There are at least three key factors related to access. The first factor is access to the pharmacist. Do you spend what seems like an eternity in the cough and cold products aisle, waiting for someone to ask you if you need some help? Do you ask the pharmacy technician if you can speak to the pharmacist, only to wait for ten or more minutes until the pharmacist can finally speak to you? The second factor is access to the pharmacy itself. Do you have to walk or drive far to get to the pharmacy? Is the pharmacy only open from 9 a.m. to 5 p.m. or is it open twenty-four hours, seven days a week? The third factor is access to the product (the medicine that the physician has prescribed). Is the pharmacy always out of stock of your favourite vitamin product and does it have an insufficient quantity of pills to fill your entire prescription?

Second, the courtesy of the pharmacist and support staff is important to patients. Does the pharmacist really care about you and look interested and engaged during the conversation or does he or she appear distracted and give you canned answers? Also related to courtesy is the timeliness of filling the prescription. As we have previously reviewed, there are legitimate reasons why every prescription cannot be filled in five or ten minutes, but most prescriptions should not take thirty minutes or more to fill, and, more importantly, if you are told the prescription will be ready in twenty minutes and when you return the prescription still is not ready without a reasonable excuse, most patients will rightly feel dissatisfied with the service they have received.

Third, the technical competency of the pharmacist and his or her staff is critical. By this we mean: Was your prescription filled correctly? Is the label legible? It probably goes without saying, but if patients experience an adverse drug event that was caused by a medication error, it is likely that they will leave the pharmacy highly dissatisfied, in addition to seeking resolution of the situation by the pharmacy. See "The Pharmacist as a Hockey Goalie?" for more details on these types of problems and what some pharmacists are doing to improve the situation.

The Pharmacist as a Hockey Goalie?

Are adverse drug events and, more specifically, medication errors a problem in community pharmacies in Canada? Unfortunately, little is known about this because presently there is no national body that collects and reports this type of information. Certainly, there have been some high-profile cases over the years of patients who received the wrong medication or wrong dose of a medication from a pharmacy and were seriously injured or died as a result. In 2008, 453 million prescriptions were dispensed in Canadian community pharmacies so even if one were to use a very conservative estimate of there being one error for every 10,000 prescriptions dispensed, that would mean 45,300 errors annually in our country!

There is a group of community pharmacies in Nova Scotia working with researchers to improve the safety of the medication-use system in their stores. This initiative is called SafetyNET-Rx, which was featured on *CTV National News*, *Canada AM*, and in other media outlets in 2009. SafetyNET-Rx involves workflow redesign to minimize the chance for an error to occur, anonymous online reporting of errors and near-errors by pharmacists, and feedback to pharmacists and pharmacy staff on trends over time. Thirteen pharmacies representing a wide variety of pharmacy types participated in the original twelve-month pilot project, and they identified approximately 1,300 of these events, which they have labelled "quality-related events." The program has expanded to 70 pharmacies in Nova Scotia as of April 2010, and may expand to other provinces in the future. The goal is to create a community pharmacy safety net where errors and near-errors will be caught before they ever reach the patient.

Of course, the community pharmacist also catches problems

with prescriptions; problems that, if left uncorrected, could harm the patient. As we reviewed earlier, pharmacists identify and resolve many drug-related problems each day without patients being aware of this fact. So, in some ways, you can think of your community pharmacist as a hockey goalie — your last line of defence, preventing medication errors and other problems from reaching you. SafetyNET-Rx helps provide the training and equipment the pharmacist needs to make as many saves as possible. For more information on SafetyNET-Rx please visit www.safetynetrx.ca.

Fourth, the clinical competency of the pharmacist is also crucial. By this we mean: Did the pharmacist provide you with good advice about your prescription? Did he or she review all the important aspects of prescription drugs, as we listed in "Things to Know and Do About Each of Your Prescriptions" on page 128.

The final factor that seems to directly impact patient satisfaction with pharmacies and pharmacy services is financial consideration. As we have reviewed, many patients in Canada pay out of pocket for the entire cost of their prescriptions while others pay a percentage of the total cost, typically called a *co-pay*. While the largest percentage of the total cost of the prescription is related to the ingredient cost of the drug itself (i.e., the price the drug manufacturer charges) and there is also a fee the wholesaler charges to the pharmacy, and the pharmacist's professional or dispensing fee. This later item is determined by contracts between the pharmacy and the third party payer (government drug plan or private insurer). Patients also price shop for lower prices of over-the-counter items in a pharmacy or items not related to health care at all, such as cosmetics, pop, and paper towels.

The *Cheers* Effect

Which factor influences patient satisfaction the most in community pharmacy? To answer this question, we can turn to an interesting study of community pharmacies in Florida. In this study, patients had received special pharmaceutical care services from their pharmacists related to managing asthma. As noted by the researchers, "patients' satisfaction was associated with the level of pharmaceutical care and their perception of the pharmacist's ability to help them with their asthma. However, personal attention from the pharmacist was most influential."[82] Thus, similar to the theme song of the 1980s television show *Cheers*, many patients want to go to a pharmacy "where everybody knows your name." This *Cheers* effect, then, seems critical, and not just to patients like Chatty Ches whom we introduced to you earlier in this chapter. The simple act of a pharmacist knowing your name, even asking about your family and other aspects of your life, strongly impacts satisfaction. It may also have a clinical impact by helping to relax patients and to form the foundation of a trusting relationship, whereby patients are more likely to confide in their pharmacist. So, ask yourself, "Is your pharmacy a place where everybody knows your name?"

Conclusion

You should now have a better understanding of the role of the community pharmacist and how to get the most out of your health-care experience in this setting. Pharmacies may offer many different services and programs, but often it takes an interested and informed patient willing to ask questions to find out about these "extras." You are now informed; hopefully you're interested in seeing what your local pharmacist can offer to you.

CHAPTER SEVEN

EXPECTING THE
UNEXPECTED

Navigating Urgent and Emergent Care

Billy Bob Balderdash is not happy. It's Friday evening and Billy Bob, an asthmatic, is about to run out of his medication. None of the family practice clinics he called after his doctor retired a few months ago are accepting new patients so he has been left an orphan of the health-care system. Finally, about to run out of his puffers, he has come to the emergency department.

Sitting across from Billy Bob is a pale-as-mashed-potatoes teenaged boy and his mother. The boy fell snowboarding about an hour ago. A nurse on the ski hill thought the laceration above his eyebrow needed to be stitched. His wrist is swollen and hurts like a son-of-a-gun; his mother suspects it needs an X-ray.

Also in the waiting room are three-year-old Emily, who has an earache, and her dad. With the family doctor's office closed for the weekend, they have also landed in the waiting room of the emergency department.

As each patient arrived, they were assessed by the triage nurse. Billy Bob wasn't happy about the questions. "I don't know what you're talking about," was his answer for many of them. "We're pretty backed up," the nurse told Billy Bob when he asked about the waiting time.

"And we never know what's coming through the door."

Hearing laughter coming from the direction of the nurses' station, Billy Bob is seething. Surely, he thinks, the staff should be looking after patients rather than cracking jokes. Then the snowboarder, who arrived after him, is taken into the treatment area. Furious, Billy Bob announces that he's leaving.

Emergency departments are where we go expecting to be cared for so we get better, not worse. Yet in 2008, a homeless man died of an overwhelming urinary infection after waiting thirty-four hours in a Winnipeg waiting room. In 2006, a Calgary woman suffered a miscarriage in front of a waiting room full of people. In a Halifax emergency department that has about 80,000 patient visits a year, the department head made national headlines on an icy day in January 2009 when, faced with patient-lined corridors and a backlog of waiting ambulances, he called a "Code Orange" — a mass casualty alert normally reserved for disasters like plane crashes. Emergency departments across the country are similarly overflowing. On the west coast, the Vancouver General alone reports almost 70,000 patient visits per year to its emergency department and Ontario's largest hospitals typically have similar numbers of visits.

So what is going on behind the double doors between the emergency department waiting room and the patient care areas to cause all that waiting? In a word, *gridlock*.

Think back to the last time you left a packed parkade after a concert or sports event. Likely you waited your turn patiently, merging with lines of traffic from other levels and vehicles backing out of parking spots. Eventually you got there, handed over your last pay cheque at the booth, and made your way home. Now imagine the same scenario but with all the exits blocked. This is the situation in many of our nation's hospitals. Normal exit routes from the emergency departments to other care areas within the hospital are blocked.

Emergency department beds, stretchers, and treatment areas are commonly occupied by patients who have been officially admitted to hospital but remain in "emerg," sometimes for days at a time, because there are no beds available for them elsewhere.

Additionally, a significant number of patients occupying inpatient beds in many hospitals no longer need hospital care. Too frail to return to independent living, these people are often awaiting placement in a long-term care facility. This number may be upward of one-third of the hospital's inpatient population. Some will wait as long as a year. As a result, admitted patients waiting for beds occupy emergency department spaces, making it difficult for staff to look after the simplest of health-care needs such as an earache, broken wrist, or prescription renewal.

Experts agree it is a myth that our emergency departments are overflowing with people who don't need care. True, many people seeking care in Canada's emergency departments could have their needs met in another location, such as a family doctor's office or a walk-in clinic. According to data from the Canadian Institute for Health Information (CIHI), 57% of individuals seeking emergency department care at 171 sites in Ontario, Nova Scotia, British Columbia, and Prince Edward Island in 2003–2004 had either non-urgent or less urgent problems (catagorized with a Canadian Triage and Acuity Score of IV or V — see page 172).[83]

In an international survey comparing Canada to the United Kingdom, Australia, New Zealand, and the United States, Canada had the highest rate of emergency department usage as well as the highest percentage of individuals reporting they waited more than two hours to be seen. Nearly one in five surveyed Canadians said they could have received care in non-emergency department settings. This number was again higher than the other four countries surveyed.[84] That doesn't mean these individuals didn't need care — they may have had no other place to access it.

Emergency department overcrowding is a symptom of a sick health-care system. A lack of beds both in the hospital and long-term care sectors is clearly a contributing factor, but other issues, such as lack of access to family physicians, are also responsible.

Public policy decisions made in the 1980s and 1990s resulted in a sharp decline in medical school enrolments. These numbers are now beginning to rebound, although it will be more than a decade before we see this turnaround translate into practising physicians. Additionally, the demographics of individuals entering the medical profession are changing. Half of Canadian medical school graduates are currently women who hit the workforce during their prime childbearing years. Physicians have one of the highest rates of burnout, stress, and suicide of any profession, and the young men and women graduating from medical school today are simply and wisely unwilling to work the gruelling hours of their predecessors.

Moreover, the characteristics of people requiring health care are different than in years gone by. Not only is our population aging, but we are more educated about options available to us and we expect more of our health-care system. If health-care spending continues to increase at current rates, some provinces predict that health budgets could consume their entire provincial budget by 2025.

Clearly, we have the makings of a perfect storm — one with a huge downspout on the doorstep of the nation's emergency departments.

There is good news, though. The sickest patients do get very prompt care in Canadian emergency departments. In the CIHI survey, the median wait time to see a physician for those patients with conditions that were immediately life-threatening was five minutes. Patients also recognize that the quality of care provided is very high. In Saskatchewan, for example, the province's Health Quality Council found 94% of patients surveyed in 2005 rated their overall quality of care in an acute-care setting as either "good," "very good," or "excellent."[85] It's moving patients through the system — unblocking the exits from emergency departments to inpatient beds, or from inpatient beds to long-term care facilities — that continues to pose challenges.

Why do people require emergency care? Being very old or very young increases your chances of seeking emergency department care. Almost half of Ontario infants and seniors older than eighty-five visited an emergency department in 2003–2004. Being poor or living in a rural community also increases your odds. Among specific health-related problems, injuries account for nearly a quarter of all visits to Canadian emergency departments. But one of the leading reasons people for emergency department visits may surprise you: A recent study suggests that one in nine visits is due to a medication-related problem.[86]

In this chapter we'll look in-depth at the issue of accessing urgent care in Canada. If you find yourself needing after-hours advice or assessment, we'll give you solid information on where to turn. Using examples from our case files we'll review typical medication-related problems that result in emergency visits and explore how you, a health-care consumer, might be able either to avoid these problems or manage them on your own. Finally, in the event you do require a trip to one of Canada's emergency departments, we'll offer practical tips on navigating your visit.

What's the Big Deal About Waiting?

As we've discussed, there are commonly delays from the time a patient is officially admitted to hospital to the time they leave the emergency department for an inpatient unit. But what does this mean for patients, besides just more waiting and perhaps a flattened backside? In a recent study of patients sixty-five years or older admitted from the emergency department in a teaching hospital in Atlantic Canada, researchers found that patients with a prolonged stay in the emergency department (more than six hours in total) were more likely to experience an adverse event while in hospital.[87] Adverse events included such things as infection after a procedure and complications related to medications. On average, those patients who had an adverse event spent twice as long in hospital. Although fewer than 3% of the patients experienced an adverse event related to medication, the tips offered in this chapter will hopefully reduce your risk of having problems.

Opening Pandora's Pill Box: Common Urgent Medication-Related Problems

Almost half of the medication-related problems that result in emergency department visits are due to side effects, or *adverse drug reactions* as health-care practitioners refer to them. But beyond this, many visits were due to the medication:

1. not being taken properly,
2. being taken in improper amounts, or
3. being ineffective for the problem.

Too much or too little — Meet Margaret and Richard
From our case files, here are two patients whose stories typify these two extremes. Consider, first, the story of Margaret.

Margaret, forty-nine, had been feeling horrible for months. She had a constant headache and was exhausted to the point that she struggled to get out of bed in the mornings. She felt overwhelmed by the demands of her job as business editor of a local newspaper and by the increasing needs of her aging parents. Her mother had Alzheimer's disease and made frequent phone calls to ask Margaret when she would be coming to visit or take her to the doctor, bank, or grocery store. As her disease progressed, she would sometimes phone to ask the same question three or four times an hour. On top of this, Margaret's son-in-law was in Afghanistan and she was often asked to care for her two young grandsons in the evening while her daughter worked or went out with friends.

Margaret felt guilty that she was often cranky and irritable with her family. "You're lucky," she told her husband. "You can get away from me. I can't get away from me." Little things — things that normally were only mildly annoying — provoked her to tears. She found herself weeping when a letter to the editor arrived critical of an article she'd written. She completely lost interest in sex, which she blamed on exhaustion as well as a fifteen-pound weight gain. Despite always being tired, she slept poorly. When she tried to fall asleep, her mind replayed an endless loop of the stressful situations facing her in the coming days. After she finally fell asleep, she almost always awoke between 2 a.m. and 3 a.m. and couldn't get back to sleep.

Margaret did some internet research and talked to friends. She wondered whether she might have a thyroid problem or a pre-menopausal hormonal imbalance. After running a series of tests, Margaret's doctor diagnosed her with depression and prescribed an antidepressant. She also suggested that Margaret see a counsellor to help her work through the stresses in her life.

After Margaret took the first few pills, she head felt lightheaded and even drowsier than she'd been previously. She called her doctor, who suggested skipping a day and then switching the pill to the evening. Margaret still felt unwell after this, so she decided to try a half a pill. Even then, the tiredness persisted, so when she had a busy day the next day she took just a quarter of a pill.

A snowstorm derailed her planned follow-up appointment with her doctor. A month passed and Margaret had been so busy she hadn't had time to either reschedule the doctor's appointment or book the appointment with the counsellor. She was contemplating stopping the medication as she was still feeling as terrible as when she'd started it.

A month after the missed appointment, Margaret's husband came home to find her in their bed. He could barely rouse her. She had taken the remainder of the bottle of pills.

Richard, seventy-one, came to the emergency department late one evening. He was nauseous and dizzy to the point he could barely stand up. He told the triage nurse and the doctor that he had "high sugar, heart problems, and trouble with his 'waterworks.'" He was taking a white pill and a pink pill in the morning and another white pill at bedtime. He didn't know their names and hadn't thought to bring them with him. His doctor's office and pharmacy were both closed and his wife, who might otherwise have been able to retrieve his medications, was visiting family in another province.

Richard was found to have a very slow heart rate and the doctor wondered whether this might be due to one of the medications he was taking. Eventually, blood tests revealed Richard had taken too much of one of his medications — one that can result in overdose even if taken in "normal" amounts. An antidote is available, but because Richard wasn't able to tell the doctor what medication he was taking, its administration was delayed. This overdose could have been fatal and Richard was very lucky that his doctor was astute enough to think to order a blood test to check levels of this uncommonly prescribed medication.

Later in this chapter we will discuss management of common medication side effects such as the drowsiness Margaret experienced on the antidepressant, but let's now look at ways in which each of them could have avoided a potentially life-threatening problem.

1. Take medications as directed — exactly as directed.

Margaret, not realizing that her depression was a potentially life-threatening problem, chose to adjust her medications based on side effects she believed she was experiencing. In all likelihood, Margaret's symptoms of worsening fatigue were due to the worsening of her depression rather than side effects of her antidepressant. Often antidepressants take several weeks to begin to work as the brain's pathways adjust. If she had discussed this with her doctor or pharmacist, Margaret might have been more willing to stick it out. Margaret's story underscores the importance of not adjusting medication doses without consulting your physician. Some doctors and pharmacists report that their patients take bits and pieces of pills in the hopes of minimizing side effects. Take it from us, these chips of flint are not going to get the job done.

2. Follow up with your physician.

Like many women in the "sandwich" generation who are providing care for aging parents as well as children and/or grandchildren, Margaret was at the bottom of her own priority list. Had she seen her doctor for the planned follow-up visit, the worsening depression

Additionally, like Speedos, medications are not one size fits all. Some individuals need a higher dose of medication than average to manage exactly the same problem — kind of like a boxer shorts version rather than a briefs. In general, if you are elderly you will need smaller doses of medication and if you are on the larger side you may need slightly more.

3. The medication is ineffective.
Sometimes medications that work very well for one person may not work at all for another. In the same way that the jeans that look awesome on your best friend may not do a thing for you, the medication that works for your heavy periods may not help her at all. While medical science helps physicians know what type of medication ought to work for an individual patient, there is no guarantee that it will. Interestingly, there is often no rhyme nor reason to explain why some individuals will improve while on a medication while others with exactly the same illness or symptoms will not. Much like the process of trying on several new pairs of jeans before finding a good "fit," there is often a process of trial and error with medications to find one that works well.

4. The diagnosis is wrong.
As we saw in a previous chapter, making a diagnosis is not always a precise science. While we don't advocate you delay seeking medical care when you need it, as a general rule of thumb the earlier in the disease you are seen, the more difficult it can be for your doctor to make a precise diagnosis. For example, if you have chicken pox and see your doctor when you have just one or two spots it may be hard for him or her to identify the nature of the rash. A day or so later, though, when you are covered in hundreds of itchy red spots, he or she can likely pinpoint the problem almost instantly. For many conditions the diagnosis becomes clearer with the passage of time.

If you don't feel better when your doctor indicated you should and you are taking the prescribed medication as recommended, call to book an appointment to have the problem reassessed. Don't try to guess whether the diagnosis is wrong, or whether your doctor is doing the start-low-and-go-slow method, or whether your Speedo is just too small — let your doctor scratch his or her head and figure it out. It's also important to note that if you feel worse or have new symptoms, don't wait for that time interval to elapse. Call and ask to be seen sooner. If you can't get in to see your doctor, calling a Telehealth network (see "Telehealth in Canada" on page 170) is another option.

You Want an Appointment When?

We see you rolling your eyes. We're telling you to call your doctor's office, but you don't think you stand a chance of getting an appointment anytime much before Armageddon. Or do you? In the 2007 National Physician Survey, 65% of family physicians indicated they offer same-day appointments for patients with urgent needs.[88] However, a Commonwealth Fund survey of patients conducted that same year found only 22% of patients could get a same-day appointment if they needed one.[89] Who's telling the truth? Drilling down further in the National Physician Survey data, physicians who are older, male, working in a solo practice and in a rural community were more likely to offer same-day appointments. Interestingly, physicians working in private offices were just as likely to have same-day appointments available as walk-in clinics (77% versus 75%, respectively).[90] We suggest calling early in the day, emphasizing that you need an urgent appointment for one problem only and making yourself available on short notice since cancellations are as common as four-year-old issues of *Readers' Digest* in most family physicians' offices.

I'll Take a Side Order

Any substance, such as a drug, that has an effect on the body's physiologic functions also has the potential to have unexpected or undesired effects on how our body functions. As mentioned, these side effects are often referred to by health-care practitioners as *adverse drug reactions*. Side effects are among the most common reasons people visit emergency departments. In this section, we'll explore how we learn about medication side effects and then review some common ones, including what you can do about them.

Side effects of a medication are identified and brought to the attention of health-care providers and consumers in several ways. In Chapter 5, we discussed how clinical trials compare the desired effect of the drug to the effects of a placebo. We also discussed how as many as 30% of people will experience a "placebo effect." This means that their illness or symptom will get better even if they receive placebo alone. Individuals participating in these trials are also monitored for side effects. This includes individuals in both the study group, those receiving the drug, and those in the placebo group. That's right — *even people who are receiving placebo report side effects*. Who knew? When the results are tabulated, side effects are compared between the two groups to determine which are more common in those who receive the drug. When a drug is first marketed, the manufacturer develops a product monograph that lists the effects of the drug as well as its known side effects. This monograph helps health-care practitioners decide whether a medication is right for a particular individual and assists them in advising and monitoring their patients.

Sometimes, though, medication side effects don't come to light until the drug has made its way onto the market.

MedEffect Canada is a Health Canada program that allows Canadians and their health-care practitioners to provide information on adverse reactions to a centralized database. This information is collected and assessed by the Canada Vigilance Program (formerly the Canadian Adverse Drug Reaction Monitoring Program) so that drugs and health-care products available in Canada can be continually monitored.

Reporting an adverse reaction to the MedEffect program can be done in one of three ways:

- by phone, toll-free, at 1-866-234-2345
- online at www.healthcanada.gc.ca/medeffect
- by completing a Canada Vigilance Reporting Form and either:
    - faxing it to 1-866-678-6789 or
    - mailing it to:
        Canada Vigilance Program
        Health Canada Address Locator 0701C
        Ottawa, ON K1A 0K9

Postage-paid labels, the Canada Vigilance Reporting Form, and the adverse drug reaction reporting guidelines are available on the MedEffect website.

Horses and Zebras — Managing Medication Side Effects

There is a saying among doctors that when you hear hoofbeats, you should think of horses, not zebras. That means when a physician is trying to diagnose a patient's illness, a common illness, rather than a rare one, is the more likely culprit.

In this section, we'll take you through common medication side effects — the horses — and tell you how you can prevent or manage many of them on your own. If the side effect you're experiencing is one of the rarer zebras that may be listed on the pharmacy printout, we suggest checking in with your physician.

If you think you are experiencing a medication-related side effect there are generally four things you can do:

1. Ride it out. Many side effects disappear in time as our body adjusts to the new medication. However, if you're having either a problem your physician or pharmacist indicated needs prompt medical attention or true allergic symptoms as outlined below, this isn't an option.

2. Reach for the phone. A call to the pharmacist or a Telehealth network to ask for advice might quickly clear up the matter.
3. Rearrange the timing or dosage of the medication after consulting your physician.
4. Return to your physician for reassessment, particularly if the side effects are so severe you can't continue taking it or you have symptoms suspicious for an allergy to the drug, such as a rash.

It is important to remember that you should almost *never* stop taking your prescription before it's finished without consulting your doctor. It seems self-evident, but it happens all the time. As we discussed in Chapter 5, there are just a handful of situations in which you should stop taking a medication without consulting the doctor — such as a suspected blood clot in your leg if you are taking the birth control pill. However, there can be serious or life-threatening risks associated with abruptly stopping some medications. Continuing to take the medication is usually the best option.

Gut Grief

Medications we swallow pass through our stomach and into our digestive tract before being absorbed into our bloodstream and delivered to the parts of the body where they do their thing. It's not surprising, then, that much of the action in terms of side effects takes place in the belly — leading to "gut grief."

Gut grief part 1: Nausea and vomiting, a.k.a. hanging on the porcelain lifesaver calling for "Ralph" and "Earl"
While almost any medication taken by mouth has the potential to cause stomach irritation and lead to nausea or vomiting, anti-inflammatory medications, steroids, some antibiotics and antidepressants, and of course chemotherapy drugs are common culprits.

If you are receiving chemotherapy, your caregivers have surely told you to expect nausea and vomiting as a side effect of your treatment and to call them if the medication they prescribed is not effective.

In the case of another medication, if you become nauseous, we suggest first checking the printed instructions to see if it can be taken with food since this may solve the problem. If you're not sure, check with the pharmacy.

Medication taken at bedtime should work its way out of your stomach by the time you wake, allowing you to sleep through any nausea. Most once-a-day medications can be taken at any time of day. For some medications, though, time of day is important; for example, many cholesterol-lowering medications work best if they are taken with the largest meal of the day and some medications may cause insomnia and so should be avoided at bedtime. In the interests of a good night's sleep, you would also likely want to avoid taking diuretics — drugs that work in part by making you urinate — on your way to bed to avoid waking up in the middle of the night with your molars floating. Before making a change like this, however, it's important to get the green light from your doctor or pharmacist.

If taking the medication with food or on the way to bed isn't in the cards and the nausea is tolerable, you can try riding it out. Like many side effects, medication-related nausea often subsides in time.

If you end up hanging onto the porcelain lifesaver more than once or twice, talk to your physician or pharmacist. For example, your doctor may suggest decreasing the medication dose temporarily to allow your body time to adjust to it. And although we're not huge fans of taking one medication to counteract the side effects of another, members of your health-care team may suggest an anti-nausea or stomach-protecting medication if it is likely you will only need the medication for a short period of time, if all of the available treatments potentially have the same side effect, or if this particular treatment is essential.

Medication that you cannot keep down because of repeated vomiting is, of course, not going to be effective. If an anti-nausea medication doesn't work, consult your doctor about prescribing something different.

Gut grief part 2: Peter Rabbit's potty

Some medications, notably narcotics (such as codeine), which are used for moderate to severe pain, can cause constipation. Prevention is key. Drink lots of water — at least six glasses a day. Beverages containing caffeine or alcohol don't count as they essentially reroute much of the fluid your colon needs to your kidneys and bladder. You may find it easier to drink enough water if you measure out your daily allotment first thing in the morning. Many people find water more palatable if it's kept at room temperature or flavoured with a little lemon, lime, or even cucumber.

Increasing fibre intake also helps, so scarf down plenty of fresh veggies and fruit and whole grains. Natural bran or psyllium can be sprinkled on anything from applesauce to zabaglione or baked into muffins or other goodies. Regular activity such as walking also helps to ward off constipation.

If these measures fail, talk to your health-care provider or pharmacist about a stool softener or laxative to keep your motor running. If you are regularly taking a narcotic for treatment of cancer-related or other chronic pain, it's best to take a stool softener or laxative on a regular basis rather than waiting for your engine to grind to a halt.

Gut grief part 3: Skip to my loo

The third part of the gut trilogy is diarrhea. This is another relatively common side effect of medications, particularly antibiotics. In Chapter 4, we describe the problem of *Clostridium difficile (C. diff.)* infection, which usually results when antibiotics kill off some bowel bacteria and allows others to proliferate and produce a diarrhea-causing toxin. This is a sobering reminder to all of us to only use antibiotics when necessary.

It is important to note, however, that not all antibiotic-related diarrhea is due to *C. diff.* While as many as 25% of people taking antibiotics develop diarrhea, most times the diarrhea is mild and corrects itself in a few days. Over-the-counter anti-diarrheal agents may be helpful for mild diarrhea. Additionally, probiotics (a food or other substance containing live micro-organisms), particularly *Lactobacillus* or *Saccaromyces boulardii*, have been shown to be effective in preventing antibiotic-associated diarrhea. Probiotics are available at many pharmacies and health-food stores.

If diarrhea develops when you are on any medication, watchful waiting may be all that is needed. If the diarrhea is severe or prolonged, a visit to the doctor is in order. This is particularly important in the very young or very old, who are at increased risk of dehydration. Medical attention is always warranted when the diarrhea is accompanied by fever, abdominal pain, or blood or pus in the stools.

Burn, baby, burn: Vaginal yeast infections

Just as antibiotics can kill off helpful bacteria in the gut, they can also kill off vaginal bacteria that help to keep yeast, a micro-organism found in the vagina, in check. If the yeast multiplies quickly, telltale symptoms of itching, burning, and vaginal discharge may occur. An over-the-counter preparation to knock off the offending yeast will usually do the trick.

Catching a few zzzz's

Sleepiness is a known side effect of many medications. Your doctor and pharmacist have likely told you if your medication might make you drowsy. If they didn't, a label on the bottle suggesting caution with driving or operating heavy machinery is a dead giveaway.

Thankfully, the sedative effect of many medications tends to wear off as our body adjusts to them. Here are a few suggestions for getting you through:

> • **If your doctor agrees it's safe to wait a few days,** start taking the medication when you don't have too much on your plate. For example, avoid starting medication that may cause drowsiness the weekend you're reshingling your roof, roto-tilling your next-door neighbour's mother's second cousin's ten-acre veg-

gie garden, and running a 10–K race. On second thought, maybe you do want to sleep through all that. We sure would.

• **For many medications that have the potential to cause sedation,** your doctor will use the principle of "start low and go slow," as outlined previously. However, it is important to work with your doctor toward taking the full therapeutic dose. Taking too little can be just the same as taking none at all. Beware those chips of flint we discussed earlier.

Dry-as-the-Mojave mouth

Many medications are non-specific in how they affect the body. That is, they may have effects on parts of the body besides the ones making us ill. Some medications, for example, might make us grow hair in funky places or give us a sense of euphoria we haven't experienced since the days we were shakin' it up to the likes of Jim Morrison or KC and the Sunshine Band. Other medications affect the autonomic nervous system, which is responsible for bowel and bladder functioning and the muscles in our eyes that control the size of our pupils. Since the autonomic nervous system also controls production of saliva, dry mouth may be a side effect.

As with other medication side effects, dry mouth tends to subside in time. Sugarless candy will usually alleviate the problem. Sugar-containing candy, besides being lousy for the waistline, tends to make the mouth even drier.

Dizzy Lizzie

Many medications have the potential to make us feel dizzy, light-headed, or shaky. Medications used to treat high blood pressure, for example, can do this by lowering our blood pressure to levels lower than our brain has become used to. Many other medications can enter the brain and lead to a "funny head" feeling, as many patients describe it. Doctors will commonly use the start-low-and-go-slow principle for these medications, and this side effect also tends to diminish in time. If, however, it's intolerable, ask the doctor whether you can take the medication on the way to bed or temporarily reduce the dose until your brain has time to adjust to it.

Medication allergies

If we had a nasty side effect from a medication, many of us would assume we're allergic to it. That's not necessarily so. A true drug allergy occurs when our body produces substances called antibodies to the drug. These antibodies trigger a series of reactions that cause a predictable pattern of symptoms such as itching, hives, wheezing, or swelling of the mouth, lips, or throat. This type of reaction, called anaphylaxis, is a true emergency and needs urgent medical attention.

Other medication effects, such as dizziness, vaginal yeast infections, or gut grief, while unpleasant, are not true allergies. They are referred to as drug intolerances.

If you believe you have symptoms of anaphylaxis, seek medical attention in an emergency department immediately. If the reaction is progressing rapidly, have someone call 911 on your behalf — don't try to drive to the hospital. Once it is confirmed that you have had a true allergic reaction to a drug, you should obtain a Medic-Alert bracelet from a pharmacy or jewellery store.

Your doctor may not be able to tell with certainty at an office visit whether you experienced a true allergic reaction to a medication. In that case, he or she may send you for allergy testing. However, this testing is not available for all medications.

Case Files: Rash Decisions

Tucker, a busy toddler, saw his family doctor one day in late October after his parents became concerned about a high fever that was accompanied by irritability and a poor appetite. His doctor saw signs of an early ear infection and prescribed an antibiotic. Less than forty-eight hours later Tucker's fever settled, but he broke out in a head-to-toe rash. His parents wondered whether Tucker might be allergic to the antibiotic and took him back to the doctor. The diagnosis: roseola — a common viral illness in toddlers that tends to make the rounds in the fall.

Tucker's case illustrates an important point: many, but not all, rashes that develop on a new medication are caused by an allergy. It is important that any rash that develops on a new medication is assessed by a physician to determine the cause. Too often, individuals are erroneously labelled as "allergic" to a medication, which can unnecessarily limit future treatment options.

In another case, Linda was prescribed an antibiotic by her doctor for treatment of a bladder infection. A few days after beginning the medication she noticed a curious rash that looked like pinpoint bruises. She called the pharmacist, who directed her to her family physician. A blood test revealed that Linda had developed dangerously low blood cell counts — a life-threatening but fortunately exceedingly rare side effect of some medications. On the advice of her physician, Linda immediately stopped taking the medication and, in time, her blood counts returned to normal. Had Linda chalked up the rash to an "allergy" and simply stopped the medication without seeing her physician, she might never have received important medical attention.

Who You Gonna Call?

So who should you contact if you think you are experiencing a medication-related problem? If the problem seems to be of a minor nature, a call to the pharmacy or a Telehealth network (see page 170) is a good place to start.

For a persistent problem, more serious symptoms including any new rash, or concerns that the medication isn't working, we suggest contacting the person who prescribed the medication. Rather than try to sort out matters over the phone, it's best to be seen in person to be sure that what you are experiencing is a side effect and not a worsening of your medical condition or a rare, serious side effect like Linda's. While your doctor may be willing to suggest a different treatment over the phone if you are experiencing a common drug-related side effect, in most instances a visit is the safest practice. If you can't get in to see your own doctor, a visit to a walk-in clinic is an alternative way to have a possible drug allergy or side effect, such as a rash, evaluated at the time the symptoms are present.

Of course health problems, like cheap underwear, have an incredible knack for creeping up at inopportune times. So, it's 7 p.m. on Friday and you think the medication the doctor prescribed for you isn't working. You've been through the printout from the pharmacy and you're taking it properly but still feel pretty rough. Or you feel miserable from what you think is a medication side effect. You don't think you can wait until your family doctor's office opens Monday morning. What do you do?

First of all, if you think you are ill enough to require immediate emergency care, trust your instincts. But if you're not sure whether you need to go, there are other options for getting health advice on a wide variety of topics, including whether you should make a trip to the emergency department:

1. Call your family doctor's office.
If you need urgent care or advice and you have a family doctor, we suggest first placing a call to his or her office. Most have contingency plans for when their patients need urgent care either during or after regular office hours. Ideally, your own physician will be available, but during office hours another doctor in the clinic, who will also have access to your health record, is the next best thing. In many areas, doctors work in collaborative care teams with a nurse or nurse practitioner who can assess and provide advice on many health problems.

After hours, some family physicians will arrange to see you at their office or, if they have hospital privileges, at the local hospital. If this is not possible, many will call a local emergency department on your behalf to let them know you are coming and to advise hospital staff of any important medical history. This doesn't mean you will be seen as soon as you arrive, but the information your doctor passes along will be helpful to members of the team who will be caring for you.

Advanced Access

Ever call your doctor's office only to be given an appointment three weeks away and by the time the appointment arrived, the problem was resolved? Guess what? It's not just you. In the late 1990s a large clinic in California found it was having similar problems. The schedule was completely full with patients booked weeks or months ahead and staff members were struggling to accommodate the patients needing to be seen urgently. The clinic went on to develop a program called Advanced Access. The premise is very simple: You are seen by your doctor on the day you call. Rather than providing the care patients needed last month (or no longer need) today, the clinic shifted instead to providing the care patients need today — today! The idea is catching on, and a number of Canadian physicians have made the transition to this scheduling model. Some use a hybrid, pre-booking a certain number of appointments such as for seniors who only can get transportation on certain days or for people with inflexible work schedules, while leaving a certain number of appointments open for patients who call that day. Physicians and patients, for the most part, give this approach two thumbs-up. If you are looking for a new doctor, it might be worth asking whether they use Advanced Access.

---

2. Call a Telehealth network.

Most Canadian provinces have programs that allow residents 24-7 access by telephone to a qualified health-care provider — usually a registered nurse. A list of programs and their phone numbers can be found below. When you call, the nurse asks a series of questions about your symptoms or concerns and then offers advice or information.

He or she may, for example, suggest self-health measures or recommend a visit to an emergency department or walk-in clinic. Alternatively, he or she may be able to provide reassurance that the problem can wait for an appointment with your regular doctor or provide phone numbers for community resources that may assist. Most Telehealth networks offer advice on a wide variety of issues, including illness or injuries, chronic health conditions, illness prevention, and healthy living.

Telehealth in Canada

British Columbia

HealthLinkBC: 811; TTY: 711. Additionally, BC Health files, fact sheets on a number of health conditions, are available at www.healthlinkbc.ca.

Alberta

HEALTHLink Alberta: 1-866-408-LINK (5465). HEALTHLink also has extensive online health information at www.healthlinkalberta.ca.

Saskatchewan

HealthLine: 1-877-800-0002

Manitoba

Manitoba Health Links: 1-888-315-9257, or 788-8200 in Winnipeg

Ontario

Telehealth Ontario: 1-866-797-0000; TTY: 1-866-797-0007

Quebec

Info-Sante: 1-514-934-0354

New Brunswick

New Brunswick Tele-Care: 1-800-244-8353

Nova Scotia

Nova Scotia Health Link: 811

Newfoundland and Labrador

Newfoundland and Labrador Health Line: 1-888-709-2929; TTY: 1-888-709-3555

Northwest Territories

Northwest Territories Tele-Care Health Line: 1-888-255-1010; TTY: 1-888-255-8211

3. Visit a walk-in clinic.

Another option for seeking urgent care is a walk-in clinic. These have become popular in Canada over the last two decades, and their role in the health-care system is hotly debated by policy-makers and physicians themselves. Advocates of walk-in-clinics say they save taxpayers millions of dollars by seeing patients who otherwise would have had a costlier visit to the emergency department. Critics, though, say that walk-in-clinics have arisen as an entrepreneurial response to fee-for-service models of paying physicians. They exist, it is alleged, only because cherry-picking shorter visits is more financially rewarding for the physicians who work there. Some say they provide fragmented care while failing to address preventive health measures, complex disease processes, and psychosocial issues that can have a profound impact on illnesses. Indeed, evidence is lacking that speedier access to care in a walk-in clinic results in better health outcomes than later care by the regular family physician. Additionally, many policy-makers remain concerned that walk-in clinics encourage people to seek care at a lower level of symptoms than is necessary.

Whatever your view, walk-in-clinics seem here to stay, at least for the time being, are incredibly convenient, and fill an important gap for individuals who don't have a family doctor or who can't access their family doctor urgently. We do suggest, however, that before going to a walk-in clinic you check with your family doctor, if you have one, as he or she may be able to provide urgent care or advice. Some walk-in clinics automatically send a copy of the doctor's notes to your family doctor, some do this only if requested, and a number don't do it at all. Records of all health-care visits are an important part of your comprehensive medical chart and you should insist that a copy of the walk-in clinic doctor's notes and any test results be sent to your family doctor.

4. Dial a doctor.

In addition, in some communities housecall services are available. Check your local phone directory to see if one is available in your area.

The Big Kahuna: Navigating the Emergency Department

At the beginning of this chapter, we looked at a typical emergency department waiting room. One of the most upsetting things for patients is when they see someone who arrived after them called in before them, especially after hours of waiting. In fact, about 3% of all visitors to emergency departments leave without being seen. What is going on?

The missing piece of the puzzle is something called *triage*, which comes from the French verb "to sort."

Arriving at the emergency department, one of the first people you encounter is the triage nurse, whose job is to listen to your symptoms, conduct a brief assessment, and assign a triage score. This score helps staff determine how urgent your illness is compared to others waiting for care and provides guidance regarding the period of time in which you should be seen. Sometimes emergency departments use computerized programs to help assign triage scores. Allied health personnel such as paramedics may also be involved in triage assessment.

Most Canadian hospitals use the Canadian Triage Acuity Score (CTAS). Subject to ongoing modifications the basics are as follows:

Level I: These patients have life- or limb-threatening conditions and need immediate resuscitative measures. Examples include a patient in cardiac arrest or an individual with severe injuries from a motor vehicle crash. Commonly, these patients arrive by ambulance, emergency department staff meets them on arrival, and a physician sees them within a few minutes. In a single-physician or small-to-medium-sized emergency department, other patients must wait until Level I patients have been treated and stabilized. Since much of this goes on behind the double doors and out of sight of the waiting room, the arrival of a Level I patient explains a seemingly inexplicable lengthy delay.

Level II: These individuals have emergent conditions that are a potential threat to life or limb and require intervention within fifteen minutes. Examples include chest pain worrisome for a heart attack, serious hemorrhage, head injury, acute psychosis, or suicidal ideation.

Level III: Level III problems could progress to a situation requiring emergency interventions. They should be seen within thirty minutes. Examples include mild to moderate asthma or abdominal pain. Moderate trauma — such as an injury to an arm or leg with an obvious deformity suggestive of a fracture — would likely be assigned a score of III. This is likely the reason the snowboarder at the beginning of our chapter was seen before Billy Bob.

Level IV: Individuals with Level IV problems have conditions that because of their degree of distress, the patient's age or potential for deterioration, would benefit from interventions or reassurance within one to two hours. They should be seen within an hour. A suspected urinary tract infection, mild abdominal pain, an earache — such as young Emily's from this chapter's introduction — or a laceration requiring suturing are common Level IV problems.

Level V: These problems, although they may be acute, have low potential for deterioration. They should be seen within two hours and many could be looked after in a non-emergency department setting, as could a number of Level IV problems. Examples include a sore throat, colds, and our friend Billy Bob's prescription renewals.

In triage, explain your symptoms clearly and concisely. Don't embellish. Seasoned triage nurses can spot trumped-up stories and it won't endear you to them. Nor will arriving by ambulance hoping this will speed you through. Triage scores are independent of the manner in which patients arrive. Be courteous. If your condition changes while you are waiting, it's important that you speak up. For example, "I can see that you're very busy here tonight and I told you when I came in that I wasn't coughing up blood but now I am." If you want to know what triage level you have been assigned, ask. Many hospitals will tell you and explain why you have been assigned that level. While hospital staff cannot give out details of other patients' conditions, some are very good at explaining the reasons for the wait, such as an unstable patient, a serious car accident, or the gridlock experienced in many hospitals.

Violence Against Emergency Department Staff

Violence directed at health-care staff is a growing concern. A 2005 survey of Canadian nurses found that more than a quarter had been assaulted on the job within the past year and almost half reported emotional abuse from a patient or patients in the same time period.[91] While Statistics Canada, in 2007, found no difference in assault rates between emergency department nurses and those working in other locations, Australian data suggest that the problem with violence against emergency department staff is almost universal, with more than 90% reporting physical intimidation or assault at some point in their career and 100% reporting they had been victims of verbal abuse.[92]

Once you are taken to a treatment area, you will be assessed by another nurse who will ask additional questions, as will the physician. In a teaching hospital, you may also be seen by nurses and/or physicians in training. Since the physician is usually the last to see the patient, they are sometimes on the receiving end of a patient's frustration. "I just told all that to the nurse. Why do I have to go through it again?" Remember that each member of the team caring for you has a slightly different role. The nuances of how you answer the question of one team member — even if it's been asked before — might reveal a wealth of important information. After all, when you are seriously ill, the more heads that are put together on your behalf, the better.

Of course, there is more waiting in the treatment room. If you need additional tests such as blood work or an X-ray, you need to wait until the tests can be completed, as well as for the results to be available. If you need to see a specialist, there is an additional wait until he or she is available. The same goes, of course, if you need a procedure completed such as a cast applied or suturing. With each of these, the timing depends on the availability of staff, whether they are attending to other patients, and how ill those patients are in relation to you. Although wait times from arrival to the time you leave the emergency department vary considerably, in the CIHI report almost half of patients completed their entire visit — from triage to seeing the doctor(s) to completing necessary investigations — in less than two hours, and half of all patients waited less than fifty-one minutes to see a physician.[93] Having a good knowledge of your medical problems and current medications will streamline your visit. For example, if you don't have a medication list, staff may need to place a call to your family physician or pharmacy. If they're busy with particularly ill patients, there may be a delay before that call can be made.

From the emergency department, you will usually be sent home, admitted for additional care, or transferred to another hospital or facility. These periods of transition from one care area to another are common places where adverse events occur. While members of the health-care team do, of course, communicate when patients are being transferred between locales, it is vitally important that you are also firmly in the loop regarding what's going on. Before leaving the emergency department for a different area of the hospital or for another hospital, make sure you (or your advocate) clearly understand what the doctor has said is wrong with you, what treatment is needed, and who will be caring for you. The doctor may, for example, tell you that you have a broken hip and are being transferred to the Please Have Mercy Hospital under the care of Dr. Sammy Sawbones for surgery to repair your hip. Sometimes you will be sent home with planned follow-up with a specialist as an outpatient. For instance, you may be told that you need to see an orthopedic surgeon regarding your fractured ankle sometime in the next few days. Be sure you know the name of the specialist you will be seeing and what to do if you don't hear from that doctor's booking staff.

If you are being sent home and told to have follow-up care with your family doctor, it is still important that you understand the diagnosis you have been given, the results of tests that were done, and the planned treatment. Emergency departments normally send a copy of the record of your visit along with any test results to your family doctor, but these may not arrive until after your appointment with him or her. Some will give you a copy of the original record of your visit, and if that's the case, guard it with your life and bring it to your follow-up visit with your own physician.

When Should You Go?

We know we're stating the obvious, but if you believe you have a medical emergency, you should proceed to the emergency department right away. We know you can't plan your illnesses, but are there times you are more or less likely to encounter longer waits.

On balance, waits tend to be shorter in smaller emergency departments. Most emergency departments report their highest number of visits from about 7 a.m. to 8 p.m. Additionally, pediatric emergency departments report increased visits in the early evening — perhaps after parents arrive home from work to an ill child. Not surprisingly, the greatest fluctuation in visit numbers occur for the less severe illnesses — the Level IV and V problems. There is also evidence to suggest that Sundays, Mondays, and holidays tend to be the busiest, regardless of the severity of the illness. Anecdotally, some of our emergency colleagues tell us that warm, sunny days, particularly those first glorious days of spring or summer, tend to be slightly quieter. However, we aren't aware that anyone has officially studied this phenomenon.

Power of Attorney for Health-Care Decisions

All of us should have a clear plan for who we would like making decisions regarding our medical care should we become incapacitated and unable to make these decisions for ourselves. Often, this is delegated to a spouse or an adult child or sibling. Make sure the person to whom you delegate this authority knows your wishes — for example, under what conditions you would or would not want to be kept on life-support machines. Ideally, these wishes should be set out in a legal document as loved ones often find it difficult to make end-of-life decisions when faced with them. If you haven't appointed a power of attorney, many provinces have legislation that allows one to be appointed from among your close family or friends.

Jumping the Queue

Does who you are or who you know make a difference in how quickly you receive care? The answer is, of course, that it shouldn't, but it happens more than most health-care professionals like to think. For example, in a 1998 Ontario study, more than 80% of physician respondents and 53% of hospital CEOs said they'd been involved in management of a patient who had received care based on factors other than medical need. The most likely patients to queue-jump were politicians, high-profile public figures, and those with personal ties to the treating physician.[94] While physicians admit they sometimes use their influence to help move friends and family along the queue, patients are also active participants in this process. A 2007 study surveyed Toronto households by telephone. Interestingly, while 95% of individuals agreed with the principle of equal access based on medical need in the emergency department, around half would call a friend who is an M.D., works for an M.D., or who is a hospital administrator if they believed circumstances warranted. In addition, 29% would give a gift or donation to the hospital if they believed it would help them to jump the queue. Sixteen percent admitted to having done one or more of these in the past.[95]

Conclusion

Canada's emergency departments are clearly pressure cookers both for the staff who work there and for the patients they care for. While many health-care problems — such as Billy Bob's prescription renewals — can clearly be looked after elsewhere, the Canadian system is such that no magic wand solutions are on the horizon. However, being an informed, in-the-loop patient and understanding how urgent care in Canada is organized and where credible information is available will go a long way toward keeping you and your loved ones healthy and improving your emergency department experience or eliminating your need to even go there at all.

CHAPTER EIGHT

HOSPITALS

Places of Healing and Harm?

Hospitals. They have been called our modern-day cathedrals. They are perhaps the most tangible part of our health-care system. Communities will rally around a hospital being threatened with closure or downsizing with passion and fervour. Large ones in urban centres may be harder to navigate than a cornfield maze. Small ones in rural communities may have less square footage than some pharmacies.

In this chapter, we will explore this complex health-care setting with the full realization that hospitals are so varied in size and scope it is difficult to capture all these nuances in a single chapter. At the same time, there are many commonalities even between a small 20-bed hospital in a remote northern community and a 1,200-bed hospital in a large urban centre. While we can't provide a user's guide for each of our nation's hospitals, we hope that you will find the information provided in this chapter to be useful to you, should you, a family member, or close personal friend be admitted to a hospital. In addition, given that hospitals are both places of healing and harm, we will provide tips and advice on how to avoid errors and other adverse events and what to do should you ever experience such an event in a hospital.

A Self-Contained City

In many ways, hospitals can be viewed as self-contained cities. Large ones may employ thousands of individuals, and have cafeterias, food courts, and restaurants, their own power-generating plants, parking garages, and mazes of interconnected buildings. It may take months for a new resident of a city to comfortably navigate around streets, locating shops and services. Similarly, it is probably not surprising that visitors and patients (and yes, even new employees) struggle to learn their way around a large hospital. After walking out of a hospital, some probably believe that the architects of these buildings create notoriously confusing layouts on purpose!

Hospitals have had an interesting evolution in Canada. Many of the first hospitals were founded by faith-based organizations and individuals such as missionaries and Jesuit priests. This is not surprising, given the Christian tradition of servicing the needs of the poor, sick, and underprivileged. Many hospitals within the Canadian public health-care system still have faith-based affiliations. Two of the more notable examples include St. Michael's Hospital, a Catholic hospital in downtown Toronto recognized for its work with the inner-city population, and the Jewish General Hospital in Montreal, recognized for its care in geriatrics and research.

Today, the majority of hospitals in Canada are public institutions, governed by an independent public board operating on a non-profit basis, receiving funding directly from the applicable provincial/territorial government. The board provides oversight and works with the hospital's senior administrative team on day-to-day control of the budget and services while provincial/territorial departments of health establish the overall budget.

The types of hospitals existing in our country have evolved over the years. A 1920s survey of hospitals in Canada included many interesting types of hospitals not seen today: isolation hospitals, tuberculosis sanatoria, hospitals for the insane, hospitals for epileptics, and leper stations.[96]

Today, there are many variations and hybrids, but, in general, hospitals can be classified into some basic groupings:

Community hospitals
These tend to be small or mid-sized hospitals in villages, towns, and cities, where a variety of procedures and surgeries are performed. However, there has been a trend toward providing fewer procedures, and many community hospitals no longer do any surgical procedures at all. It is a real area of concern in many communities. While there is concern that a certain volume of services is needed to allow for appropriate expertise, it leaves these small hospitals without trained staff in the event of certain medical situations occurring. The communities in which these hospitals are located are typically very involved in fundraising and other hospital activities, and the hospital can be a source of pride or "bragging rights" for the community, even helping to attract potential employers or residents.

Tertiary hospitals
These typically handle complex surgeries or procedures such as an organ transplant or open-heart surgery. Patients are often referred to these facilities by their physician or a community hospital or are transferred directly from another hospital, sometimes via ambulance or helicopter. Some also distinguish tertiary hospitals from another category called *quaternary hospitals*, which provide sub-specialty services, such as advanced trauma care.

Regional hospitals
These are a hybrid between community and tertiary hospitals but are usually more similar in function to community hospitals.

Specialty hospitals
These are a subset of tertiary hospitals that focus on a single aspect of care or a specific patient population. Common examples of specialty

hospitals include maternity, pediatric, rehabilitation, and mental health hospitals.

Teaching hospitals
These are hospitals where medical and allied health (nursing, pharmacy, other) students receive training in a direct patient-care environment. Teaching hospitals are often research hospitals as well, participating in clinical trials (see Chapter 10) and in other types of research.

A single hospital may, in fact, fit into several of these categories, adding to the confusion of trying to classify hospitals. So, it is possible for a hospital to be classified as tertiary, specialty, teaching, and research all at the same time.

Most hospitals in Canada are public, and yet there is a role for private insurance even in public institutions. For example, private insurance can enable a patient to receive a private or semi-private (shared with one other patient) room, as opposed to a ward room (typically shared with three other patients). Public hospitals will sometimes receive funding from private insurance companies to do work on their behalf (such as for the Workers' Compensation Board). Private hospitals are rare but also exist in Canada. Read "Shouldice Hospital: Unlike Any Other" to learn more about one of the more unusual examples of a private, specialized hospital in Canada.

Shouldice Hospital: Unlike Any Other
While most hospitals in Canada are either community or tertiary-care hospitals, are "public," and receive their operating budgets from a provincial or territorial government, there are some exceptions. One of the more interesting of these exceptions is the Shouldice Hospital in Thornhill, Ontario, just north of Toronto. It was established by Dr. Edward Earle Shouldice in the 1940s.

This hospital is unusual for several reasons. First, it is a privately owned and run hospital, although residents of Ontario with a valid health card are covered for their hospital expenses by the provincial government. Second, the hospital specializes in just one procedure: hernia repair. The hospital has developed an expertise in this area, resulting in a high success rate that is recognized worldwide. Third, the hospital more closely resembles a country club than a typical hospital. This allows patients to feel more relaxed and to recover and heal in a pleasant environment. And finally, Shouldice's approach to care is unparalleled. For example, the hospital hosts an annual patient reunion party, typically attracting more than 1,000 former patients, which is held at the swanky Royal York Hotel in downtown Toronto. The event was first held in 1948 by Dr. Shouldice, providing him an opportunity to thank his patients and to do a checkup examination. A second example of Shouldice's unique approach to care is exemplified by its exercise regimen for their patients. The patients, typically men in their fifties to seventies, participate in an aerobics class in an attempt to get them moving and active post-surgery.

Others have recognized Shouldice's innovative methods and the hospital has been featured on *CTV National News* and in a Harvard Business School case study.[97] This "competence plus care" approach has caused some to wonder that if it can be done for hernia repair, can this delivery model for health care be replicated for other conditions?

Another aspect of the evolution of hospitals in Canada is that it is becoming increasingly difficult to tell where the "hospital" starts and stops. For example, some hospitals have clinics located near or within the main physical structure of the hospital, and often many procedures are conducted without requiring an overnight stay, or admission, of the patient. Furthermore, many diagnostic services formerly conducted exclusively within the walls of a hospital, such as magnetic resonance imaging (MRI), are now offered in clinic settings. Some of these services are being provided in private, for-profit clinics. Many hospitals have an outpatient pharmacy located onsite that may be part of a national community pharmacy chain. In some provinces, hospitals are part of larger regional health authorities, which offer many community-based health services such as public health nurses who make home visits to mothers who have recently had a baby. Sometimes hospital-affiliated services may be moved out of the hospital and to a clinic setting in another location altogether. For example, staff in an outpatient mental health clinic could be employed by a hospital and yet the clinic could be located across town from the hospital. This blurring of the boundaries of hospital care is expected to continue into the future, especially as new technologies develop, such as those that enable surgeries to be performed at one site but led by a surgical team located at a remote location.

The largest single category of health-care spending is on hospitals, and the hospital "slice" of the health-care spending "pie" has decreased over time. In 1975, 44.7% of all health-care spending in Canada was related to hospitals. By 2009, this had decreased to 27.8%. Yet, despite this decrease in the slice of the pie, the size of the health-care pie has grown greatly over time so we are spending more than ever on hospital care. In 2009, $51 billion of health-care spending was attributable to hospitals. This includes construction and renovation costs, operating costs, the salaries of hospital professionals and staff, as well as the costs of drugs given, laboratory tests performed, and equipment purchased and used within the hospital setting.[98]

Although we are spending more than ever on hospitals, it does not mean that all hospitals have adequate staff and equipment, nor are they all new, gleaming, modern medical facilities. In many communities across Canada, particularly in rural areas, hospitals are outdated and face pressure simply to provide adequate access to care for the patients they serve. "Hospitals in Crisis?" describes the situation in one such hospital in the interior of British Columbia.

Hospitals in Crisis?

As we discussed earlier, the issue of outdated hospitals in Canada is one that usually attracts the attention of both the general public and the media. To be fair, in recent years across Canada, there has been considerable investment in constructing new hospitals and in updating and modernizing existing facilities. Even when new hospitals are constructed, however, typically there is still a sizable portion of fundraising for equipment and other essentials that must be raised by the local community. Regrettably, other hospitals have languished behind with outdated facilities. One of these hospitals that attracted media attention in the past is the Kootenay Lake Regional Hospital in Nelson, B.C.

In 2000, the Canadian Press, *Maclean's* magazine, and other media outlets featured articles describing the condition of this facility, built in 1954. Dr. Philip Malpass, an internist at the hospital, described the conditions at that time, saying, "We've got a facility here that's crumbling around us" and "It's an unsupportable situation . . . I'm getting desperate." He went on to describe the dated X-ray machine: "We're not even sure it's safe. We don't know how much radiation loss is occurring and whether the staff and myself are being exposed to excess radiation." Dr. Malpass also discussed issues with the autoclave, which sterilizes the hospital waste: "I can't tell you how long ago it broke down because we're not certain. We're not certain how long the specimens were being inadequately sterilized." Problems were not restricted to old or malfunctioning equipment; one of the hospital nurses couldn't recall a new nursing position in the eleven years she had worked there and spoke to the significant workload on the nursing staff: "This is my sixth 12-hour shift in a row." Dr. Malpass offered a warning about the hospital: "Somebody is going to die. And who's going to be responsible for that?"[99]

So, what happened to the Kootenay Lake Regional Hospital? On

April 9, 2009 — almost nine years after these articles about the hospital were written — the British Columbia Ministry of Health Services announced a $15.3 million renovation for the facility.[100]

On December 14, 2009, construction finally started. The renovations are expected to be completed by spring or summer 2011.[101] The Kootenay Lake Regional Hospital may not be representative of other hospitals in Canada, but certainly many others have shared the problems of overworked medical and nursing staff, antiquated equipment, and challenges in fundraising and in updating facilities. While our country contains some of the most modern and expensive medical facilities in the world, many other hospitals are struggling just to keep their doors open.

Given that many hospitals face pressures to provide reasonable access to high-quality and safe health care, you may be wondering who is responsible for watching over our nation's hospitals. As we have reviewed in this chapter, the vast majority of Canadian hospitals are operated as private, non-profit entities run by community boards. At a national level, there is a special role for an organization called Accreditation Canada (www.accreditation.ca). This is a not-for-profit independent organization that reviews hospitals, assessing them according to national standards of excellence. In recent years, it has placed more emphasis on patient safety and on how hospitals pro-actively try to prevent adverse events and how hospitals deal with adverse events when they do occur. It uses teams of onsite surveyors, typically health professionals, who visit hospitals to observe processes of care and procedures and interview front-line health workers.

A second national organization, the Canadian Institute for Health Information (CIHI) (www.cihi.ca), also plays a significant role. Canada's provincial and territorial governments share their healthcare data with this organization, and then CIHI analyzes the data and produces reports and other publications on issues related to access, affordability, quality, and safety. One of its more recent efforts has been the creation of a publication that reports *hospital standardized mortality ratios* (HSMRs). What does this term mean? Essentially, HSMRs compare the actual number of deaths in a hospital to the national average and attempt to take into consideration other factors such as the types of patients admitted to the hospital (i.e., it does not penalize tertiary hospitals for having more acutely ill patients). The whole report can be downloaded for free from the CIHI website if you are curious about the performance of your local hospital.[102] Be warned, though; one major limitation of this report is the small number of hospitals currently included in the report (less than eighty — roughly one-tenth of all the hospitals in Canada).

Now that we have provided a general introduction to hospitals, we are going to walk you through the journey of a patient, Bryce, from admission to discharge.

You've Been Admitted to a Hospital — Now What?

Bryce is finally alone in his hospital bed for the first time. It has been a whirlwind of a day. In fact, the past twenty-four hours are a blur.

It all started yesterday when he fell on some ice while shovelling the snow outside his home. His wife, Pam, had told him that at age sixty-three, he should really cut down on outside activities and just pay one of the neighbourhood children to clear the snow from their driveway and walkway in the winter. But Bryce was too proud to allow a ten-year old do his work and so he insisted on doing it himself. Of course, it was easy for his wife to tell him "I told you so" after the accident. As soon as Bryce fell on the ice, he knew something wasn't right. A trip to the emergency department confirmed it was a hip fracture, and after more tests he was told that he would need a total hip replacement. He would be admitted to the hospital right away, with surgery scheduled for the next day.

After his wife helped him with the admission paperwork and to get settled into his semi-private room, a floodgate of people in white lab coats seemed to come in and out of his room for the next three hours. There was the surgeon, Dr. Ryan, who came in and gruffly introduced himself, told Bryce what to expect the next day with the surgery, and then quickly left. There was his first nurse, Stacy, who helped interpret what Dr. Ryan had just told him. There was the medical student who looked like he was nineteen — was his name Dr. Newman? — and asked him a seemingly endless list of questions. Then, nurse Stacy asked many of the same questions again about an hour later. Next, a pharmacist named Richard asked him about his medications — don't any of these people talk to each other? Bryce wondered. He also recalled Bartley, the technician who asked if he wanted his little TV attached to his bed hooked up. He eventually lost count of the number of people who came in to ask questions, to poke his skin with a needle, or to do both. And — ah yes — there was the person who brought in his dinner, if you called it a meal, given his food restrictions because of tomorrow's surgery.

At least now he is finally alone. He can't sleep, though. Part of it is anxiety about tomorrow's surgery. Part of it is the feel of the hospital gown he is wearing. Man, he misses his favourite PJs. Part of it is just being in a new, strange environment. He can hear the nurses talking outside his room — are they talking about him? He can hear the strange noises of the hospital. Most of all, he can hear the groaning from his roommate, who had total hip replacement surgery this morning and is obviously not completely free of pain. Finally, he decides to say a quick prayer and ask the good Lord for a speedy recovery and, most of all, a quick return back home.

You've Entered the Twilight Zone

Those who work in a hospital eventually become accustomed to their workplace. But for patients — especially those who have not spent time in a hospital previously — everything about a hospital seems to feel and look bizarre. There are many commonalities across hospitals including schedules, the types of individuals who work there, and things that can best be described as a hospital culture. We will take a few minutes to explore this very unique health-care setting and its culture and what you can expect if you are admitted to a hospital.

Deciphering the hospital schedule

As Bryce will soon discover, there are predictable peaks and valleys of activity in hospitals. Hospitals use twenty-four-hour military-type time and have standardized times for everything from when meals are distributed to when the nursing staff administers medications. Morning tends to be the time with the greatest activity, as many surgeries are planned for this time of day and often there is a buzz of activity associated with discharging patients from the hospital. A key activity in the morning in many hospitals is the *medical rounds* (see "Making the Rounds" to learn more about this cornerstone of medical practice in the hospital setting). Visiting hours for the family and friends of patients tends to be in the late morning and late afternoon to early evening, with a rest time for patients after lunchtime. In many hospitals, there is a nursing shift change around 7:00 p.m. or 7:30 p.m., and typically things quiet down considerably from about 8:30 p.m. through to the early morning. Visiting hours may be much more restricted for critically ill patients such as those in intensive care units (ICUS) and liberalized for those who are dying. They may also be restricted if there is a serious communicable disease circulating in the community — such as during a flu pandemic — in order to reduce the chance of illness spreading in this vulnerable population.

Making the Rounds

Medical rounds have been a staple of the hospital culture in most western countries for decades now. Where did they begin and what do they involve? The term originated at Johns Hopkins Hospital in Baltimore, Maryland, where medical students received lectures in a round room. The medical faculty stood in the middle of the room at the ground level with medical students on the levels above them, looking down, leaning over a circular handrail, interacting with the faculty about patient cases. Today, the term is associated with the activity of the physician circulating to his or her patients, visiting them in their rooms, checking on their status, and perhaps prescribing new medications or making other changes to their care plan. In large teaching hospitals, it is not uncommon for a room full of individuals to join the lead physician on the rounds. These individuals may include nurses, pharmacists, occupational therapists, physiotherapists, respiratory therapists, social workers, and others. In teaching hospitals, typically medical residents and students from all health professionals join in on the medical rounds too. While some patients may question the need for so many students to be part of the medical rounding team, being involved in the actual decision-making about patients is an important part of the training of these individuals.

From the patient's perspective, it may feel intimidating to have several individuals, all wearing various colours and lengths of lab coats, staring at you and taking notes on clipboards or on handheld devices. This is an opportune time, though, to ask questions about your care, procedures, medications, or the timeline for discharging you from the hospital. Because this is the one time of day when many of the key individuals involved in your care are together in one place, decisions can be made quickly.

The hospital maze

While the size and scope of hospitals vary dramatically, there are some consistent elements in their design and architecture. The patient care units, sometimes called *units* or *floors* by health-care professionals, are where the patient rooms are located, usually organized by patient type or condition. For example, some hospitals have a general or internal medicine unit, an oncology unit, a maternity unit, a pediatrics unit, and so on. Patient care units are also divided by the level of acuity (the medical stability) of the patients. In intensive care units (ICUs), one will find the patients who are most acutely ill, and these units have the highest ratio of health professionals to patients. Common examples of patients found in ICUs are those waiting for, or recovering from, heart surgery or newborn babies who are born prematurely. At the lower end of acuity are rehabilitation units, where patients may be learning how to regain bodily functions following a stroke and are receiving care from therapists, or units where patients are simply waiting for a bed in a long-term care facility to open up so they can leave the hospital.

At the centre of patient care units is the nursing station. This is the hub of activity in a unit, where the patients' charts are accessed. The medical chart is the place where health professionals document the progress of the patient, where lab test results are stored, and where physicians write orders. The medications for the patients on the unit are typically located in a room near the nursing station, where there is typically also a break room for the nurses. Many units are designed in an X or Y shape, with the nursing station in the middle. If you are visiting a unit for the first time looking for a particular patient, this is where you would ask where to find your friend or relative.

The other patient care and support areas of a hospital are located elsewhere throughout the hospital, sometimes only reachable via a winding maze of corridors, hallways, and elevators. These include food services and the cafeteria, the emergency department, operating rooms, the pharmacy, the laboratory, the power-generating area, administration offices, diagnostic equipment such as MRIs and CT scans, the chapel, the supplies area, and many other areas, including the favourite among visitors, the omnipresent gift shop. Many hospitals also have a "secret" communication mode that connects many of these areas — a pneumatic tube system. Via this system, orders and other things such as small medical supplies or medications can be fit into large capsule-shaped devices (which are about a foot in length) and quickly transported to another area in the hospital.

When one considers all these various areas and the fact that some hospitals have merged together, been renovated or built in stages over a period of several years, it is probably not too surprising that many have a confusing layout. There are some innovative approaches that attempt to lessen the confusion rather than just assigning a different paint colour to each floor. The Credit Valley Hospital (www.cvh.on.ca) in Mississauga is an example of a hospital that has received recognition for its patient-friendly architecture and layout. Another noteworthy example is the hospital in the Disney-planned community of Celebration City, Florida (www.celebrationhealth.com).

Who are all these people?

Another aspect of hospital culture to which Bryce has already been exposed is the untold number of people who wear lab coats of different lengths, health professional clothing *(scrubs)* of different colours and patterns, suits, and other attire. It is true that in some communities, the hospital may be one of the largest employers, with an army of employees and physicians working in the patient care units as well as in the other support areas we have mentioned. In general, these individuals can be divided into four categories.

Administrators

These individuals can be further subdivided into senior administration and mid-level managers and supervisors. The senior administrative team of a hospital typically consists of a chief executive officer (CEO), who reports to the board and who works with the following individuals: a chief operating officer, chief medical officer, chief financial officer, vice-president of patient care, and others. Hospitals are divided administratively into departments, often according to a health professional discipline or support service. For example, hospitals have a pharmacy department, led by a director of pharmacy, and, in larger hospitals, this person is supported by associate and assistant directors of pharmacy, clinical coordinators, and supervisors. These individuals oversee pharmacists, pharmacy technicians, pharmacy residents, and pharmacy students. Some hospitals use a management model called *program management* where the financial resources of a given patient care unit are managed together, cutting across different health disciplines. Some small hospitals in Canada have far fewer administrations. For example, there are some pharmacy departments that only consist of a single pharmacist, who has both administration and patient care functions, and a technician or two.

Sometimes you will hear researchers or commentators complain about financial waste in health care and question why so many administrators are needed. In the early to mid-1990s, there were sizeable cuts to middle management in health care, and some hospitals are struggling to cope with these cuts yet today. While it is easy to take pot-shots at administrators, they do play a critical role in overseeing the quality and safety of care, in financial management, and working with organizations such as Accreditation Canada.

Medical staff

Physicians are a key part of any hospital. In addition to their patient care responsibilities, most doctors also have administrative duties and serve on committees. There is a wide variety of medical staffing models in hospitals across Canada that are hard to concisely summarize here, but we will review some of the most common models.

As organizations, hospitals have a review process whereby they grant permission for physicians to see patients in their facility, order tests, and perform other functions. This is called *hospital privileges*. Typically in rural and smaller hospitals, the patient's own family physician has hospital privileges, and this person may be the main physician overseeing their own patient's care while they are hospitalized. In some communities, the duty of seeing patients in the hospital rotates around a group of physicians, all of whom have hospital privileges. In tertiary and specialized hospitals, typically the patient's own family physician will not see the patient in the hospital and, in many cases, may not even be aware their patient has been hospitalized until they receive a discharge report from the hospital several days or weeks later. However, in communities of all sizes, there has been a gradual trend away from family physicians providing care for their patients while they are in hospital. In some hospitals, the care may be provided by a specialist; this is often the case in larger teaching hospitals. In many places, a new type of physician, the *hospitalist*, has emerged. Hospitalists are usually family doctors by training, and their role is to provide care to patients whose family physician does not have hospital privileges. In many cases, several physicians are involved in the care of the patient. An orthopedic surgeon may conduct Bryce's surgery and ensure that he's healing appropriately, while his diabetes may be monitored by his family physician or an internal medicine specialist. However, in all cases, one physician should be designated as the "Most Responsible Physician;" the "go to" person when nursing, other staff members, or family have questions for the medical team. In Bryce's case, his care is directed by an orthopedic surgeon, Dr. Ryan, and his team. In teaching hospitals, medical residents and students play a large role in patient care and may well be the primary physicians with whom a patient interacts.

Health professional staff
A wide variety of health professionals work in the hospital setting. The most visible of these, of course, are nurses. Their importance cannot be overstated; as we reviewed in Chapter 2, a risk factor for self-reported health-care errors is perceived lack of nursing staffing. Nurses have both a rewarding and challenging career. Their career is rewarding as they can make strong bonds with patients and see how their interactions with patients have a positive impact on quality of life. At the same time, excessive workloads, shift work, and other workplace stressors can lead to burnout and job dissatisfaction among nurses.

A given patient may have two to three primary nurses during a twenty-four-hour period, depending on the number of shift changes by the nursing staff. In addition, other nurses may briefly take over a patient's care, for example, while the patient's assigned nurse is on a lunch break or with another patient. Our advice is to make it a priority to get to know your nurses and interact with them. Don't be afraid to ask questions about what your nurse is doing or if you require something. In many ways, your nurse is your intermediary between you and your physician, given that often you may only see your physician during the medical rounds in the morning.

It is also important to realize that while your nurse is there to help you, he or she is also responsible for the care of several other patients. The number of patients that a nurse oversees is dependent primarily on the acuity level of the patients; in an ICU setting, the ratio of nurses to patients may be 1:1 while on a general medicine unit the ratio may be four or five patients for each nurse. A question asked by many patients is "Why do I have one nurse one day and the next day that same nurse is assigned to a different patient?" The nursing manager assigns nurses to specific patients, and while there is an attempt at creating some continuity between specific nurses and specific patients, this is not always possible. One other consideration is that the hardest time of the day to reach your nurse is during shift overlap. This is usually a thirty-minute period when the nurses about to end their shift report on the status of their patients to the incoming nurses.

Support staff
The final group of individuals who work at hospitals are the support staff. These include clerical staff, medical records personnel, housekeeping, food services, and volunteers. Many of these individuals work behind the scenes and may never be seen by a patient during their hospitalization, yet their role is critical. For example, the staff working in food services must create customized meals for specific patients to be delivered at specific times, while also preparing meals for hospital staff and visitors. Conversely, other types of support staff, such as the housekeeping staff, sometimes make personal connections with patients and share facts with the nursing staff as

they are in the patient rooms quite often.

We could easily fill pages in this book describing the specific roles of key individuals in the hospital setting. Instead, we will take this opportunity to single out the important role of one individual — the unit clerk. These individuals are the eyes and ears of a patient care unit. Often they are responsible for letting nurses, pharmacists, and other health professionals know when a physician has written a new order, letting nurses know when one or more of their patients has pressed a call-bell on their bed and wishes to speak to their nurse, and they interact with the family and friends of patients. Needless to say, these individuals must be skilled at multitasking. In some patient care units, the unit clerk may only be present during the day shift while nurses assume these duties during the night shift.

Privacy, Please

One aspect of hospital culture that has caused concern for Bryce and that many patients dread is the lack of privacy. Some patients may even feel dehumanized through this process. But hopefully patients will recognize that the potential benefits of surgery or other procedures far exceed inconveniences such as lack of privacy.

Processes Upon Processes of Care

It is two days after his total hip replacement surgery and Bryce is doing quite well. Dr. Ryan has assured him that the surgery went smoothly and his nurses have been some of the kindest people he has ever met. He has been groggy and sleepy much of the time and vaguely recalls conversations with his wife, Pam, and their daughter, Julia. Today, the physio staff got him out of his bed and he took his first assisted walk down the hall. It was difficult to do, but he was energized by the sense of accomplishment.

It has been an hour since the walk and he is starting to feel quite a bit more pain in his hip. He presses his call-bell. Stacy, his favourite nurse, happens to be his nurse today and she enters his room a couple of minutes later. She tells him that he is already taking medications for pain but that perhaps she could contact the medical resident currently on duty to see if an additional medication could be prescribed or if the dosage could be increased.

Back at the nursing station, Stacy asks the unit clerk to track down the medical resident via the hospital paging system. A few minutes later, the resident comes up to the nursing station, chats with Stacy about Bryce, and writes an order for a new medication. This medication is not readily available in the medication room behind the nursing station. The unit clerk pulls a carbon copy of the newly written medication order from Bryce's medical chart and sends it via the pneumatic tube system to the pharmacy, which is located in the basement of the hospital, four floors down. There, a pharmacy technician pulls the order out of the pneumatic tube and enters the order into the pharmacy computer system. A pharmacist checks the order for accuracy and for drug-related problems. He is concerned about an interaction with one of the other medications Bryce is taking and pages the medical resident to clarify this. Five minutes later, the resident calls him and together they agree to change the order to a different medication. In the IV room of the pharmacy, another technician now prepares this medication and the pharmacist double checks the final product. Another technician takes the medication and delivers it back up to the patient care unit and hands it to the unit clerk. By this time, Stacy is with another patient, and the unit clerk tries to figure out which patient Stacy is helping. She finally tracks Stacy down and five minutes later Stacy comes to the nursing station to pick up the IV bag and goes into Bryce's room to hang the bag. Remarkably, this whole process has only taken fifty minutes and almost immediately Bryce feels better and falls asleep.

This scenario is fictitious, of course, but it is based on the process of getting a new medication to patients in some hospitals in Canada. The process of getting the right medication to the right patient is only one of hundreds of care processes that occur in hospitals every day for a given patient, with many of the processes occurring concurrently. Often, as was the case with our medication example, there are numerous handoffs between different individuals (there were at least twelve handoffs in our example with Bryce). As we will discuss later in this chapter, each handoff is an opportunity for an error to occur.

One method that some hospitals are now using to try to track these processes of care and that also attempts to standardize the processes is something called a *clinical practice guideline, care map,* or *care plan.* For example, for many orthopedic surgeries, there may be a care map that outlines all the essential things that should be performed before, during, and after surgery. Often, the care map is posted on a bulletin board in the patient's room so all health professionals and staff entering the room can easily check it. Care maps are usually very specific, describing things that should be done on an hourly basis. While there is the need to account for differences in individual patients and to make exceptions to care maps, overall, a care map is an excellent way to ensure that key parts of a patient's treatment plan are not forgotten or missed. In a survey of 272 Canadian hospital executives and managers, clinical practice guidelines were cited as being the best way to optimize the use of medications.[103]

Places of Healing

In these past few pages, as we've reviewed issues with culture and the complexity of care in hospitals, one thing that can be easily overlooked is the enormous value of hospitals. We may take it for granted, but hospitals are wondrous places where some amazing things occur, such as lives that are saved, people receiving new hearts, and stroke patients learning how to walk again. The advances of modern medicine, health-care technology, informatics and the abilities of highly skilled health professionals have enabled the impossible to become possible in health-care today. From world-renowned hospitals such as the Hospital for Sick Children (Sick Kids) in Toronto to local community health centres and hospitals, there is much to be proud of in Canada.

Nonetheless, even with these glowing attributes of hospitals, most Canadians have a love–hate relationship with their hospitals. What do we mean by this?

Canadians love their hospitals. As we discussed previously in this chapter, hospitals are a source of civic pride and some Canadians even base their decisions on where to live partially on proximity to a hospital. Hospitals are the single largest expenditure of the single largest budget item (health care) of all provincial budgets.

Canadians also hate their hospitals. We may not hate the actual physical structure, but certainly there are many who dislike the smells and sounds of hospitals, try to avoid them as a patient at all costs, and, if admitted, desire to leave the place as soon as possible.

A few quotes capture some of the essence of this side of the relationship.

I know how I do not want to die. I do not want to die in a hospital bed, hooked up to a multitude of tubes that are connected to machines that breathe for me, produce urine on my behalf, or beat in place of my heart. I have had a great life, and I am enjoying the best years of my life. I want to preserve the remainder of it as long as I can, but not at any cost.

— Lofty L. Basta, *A Graceful Exit* [104]

There were other tests, some of which seemed to me to be more an assertion of the clinical capability of the hospital than of concern for the well-being of the patient.

— Norman Cousin, *Anatomy of an Illness* [105]

One challenge that many patients face when hospitalized that they may not have expected upon admission is keeping a positive attitude. It can be easy for patients to be overwhelmed by the hospital culture. Lack of privacy, a strange environment, being in discomfort, nervousness about procedures, and uncertainty about outcomes — these are all things that Bryce faced in our example and that many patients face on a daily basis.

This may be true, but hospitals are also places of healing and hope. As "A Window into the Soul" demonstrates, sometimes it is patients themselves who give each other hope.

A Window into the Soul

In his book *Developing the Leader Within You*, author and leadership expert John Maxwell provides a summary of an essay by G.W. Target called "The Window." It is a powerful essay, showcasing the impact one man made on his roommate in a hospital room.

Both men were seriously ill and though they were not allowed much diversion — no television, no radio, or books — their friendship developed over months on conversation. They discussed every possible subject in which they both had interest or experience, from family to jobs to vacations, as well as much of their own personal histories.

Neither man left his bed, but one was fortunate enough to be next to the window. As part of his treatment he could sit up in bed for just an hour a day. At this time he would describe the world outside to his roommate. In very descriptive terms he would bring the outside world inside to this friend, describing to him the beautiful park he could see, with its lake, and the many interesting people he saw spending their time there. His friend began to live for those descriptions.

After a particularly fascinating report, the one man began to think it was not fair that his friend got to see everything while he could see nothing. He was ashamed of his thoughts, but he had quite a bit of time to think and he couldn't get this out of his mind. Eventually his thoughts began to take their effect on his health, and he became even more ill, with a disposition to match.

One evening his friend, who sometimes had difficulty with congestion and breathing, awoke with a fit of coughing and choking and was unable to push the button for the nurse to come to his aid. The frustrated, sour man lay there looking at the ceiling, listening to this struggle for life next to him, and doing nothing.

The next morning the day nurse came in to find the man by the window dead.

After a proper interval, the man who was so eager to see out that window asked if he could be moved, and it was quickly done. As soon as the room was empty, the man struggled up on his elbow to look out the window and fill his spirit with the sights of the outside world.

It was then he discovered the window faced a blank wall.[106]

Places of Harm

Another side to the hospital experience for many patients that is being increasingly recognized by clinicians, researchers, and policymakers includes adverse events that may occur during the course of hospitalization. All health-care interventions — whether a surgical procedure, diagnostic test, or medication — have the potential to harm. Yet Canadians don't enter the doors of a hospital expecting to be harmed rather than healed during their stay. As you may recall from Chapter 2, adults in Canadian hospitals each year experience approximately 185,000 adverse events, so this is not an insignificant problem.[107]

A study published in late 2009 helped to quantify the costs associated with these events. In this study, 140 seniors who experienced an adverse event during their hospitalization were compared to 842 seniors who did not experience an adverse event during their hospitalization. Those who experienced an adverse event stayed in the hospital roughly twice as long (20.2 days versus 9.8 days), resulting in an extra 1,400 days these patients spent in the hospital. It likely goes without saying, but these are hospital beds that could have been used by other patients. The total average cost of hospitalization was approximately $7,500 higher in the patients who experienced an adverse event, costing the health-care system an extra $650,000. If these extra costs were realized in the 140 patients in this study, the overall financial impact across our country from the 185,000 annual adverse events cannot be easily overlooked. As the authors of this study concluded, "Adverse events exact an enormous personal cost to patients and a substantial financial cost to the healthcare system."[108]

In the United States, both the Medicare and Medicaid programs stopped paying for the extra costs caused by preventable adverse events in fall 2008.[109] Up until then, hospitals could bill these programs for the extra costs associated with the additional care that patients who experienced an adverse event required. Under the new system, had Bryce been a Medicare or Medicaid patient in the United States and experienced deep vein thrombosis or pulmonary embolism (two types of blood clots) following his hip replacement procedure, this would have been deemed to have been a preventable adverse event and his hospital would not have received payment for the extra costs associated with his care. To date, there have been no similar initiatives in Canada to restrict funding to hospitals when these types of events occur.

Adverse drug events and medication errors
Adverse drug events, including medication errors, can lead to hospital admissions and can occur at any point after patients have been admitted. In one Vancouver hospital, roughly one out of every nine emergency department visits was related to an adverse drug event.[110]

These patients were also more likely to be admitted to the hospital and, once admitted, stayed longer than patients who did a not have an adverse drug event-related emergency department visit. In a survey of hospital executives and managers, *medication errors* was tied for first place in a list of most important drug-related issues facing hospitals.[111] Let's take a closer look at a couple of studies that have explored the issue of adverse drug events in the hospital setting to see if we can observe any themes or trends.

The first study was set in a medical/surgical ICU in Tucson, Arizona. In this study, the ICU was observed for 16.5 consecutive days by the research team, in an attempt to detect adverse drug events and medication errors. In all, 132 "clinically important" medication errors were observed. In perhaps what is the most alarming result to come out of this study, there was one error for every five doses of medication administered to the patients over the course of the study! The most common problems observed in this study were drug omission (the drug was not given to a patient and it should have been given), the wrong dose of the drug was given to the patient, and the wrong drug was administered. The researchers then tried to determine the cause of these problems. The top causes of problems were identified as being lack of drug knowledge by the prescriber, slips and memory lapses, and error in drug identification (i.e., the nurse thought she was giving the correct drug but didn't check it adequately).[112]

In another study at a hospital in Halifax, Nova Scotia, the focus was on documentation. More specifically, the researchers in this study compared the handwritten medication order by the physician in the patient's chart to the entry in the pharmacy department's computerized prescription profile to the handwritten entry in the nursing medication administration record on the patient care units. The research team reviewed 1,424 medication orders in 197 patients, comparing the documentation between these three sources of information and looking for discrepancies. Slightly more than one out of every eight medication orders contained at least one discrepancy, with 61% of patients having at least one discrepancy. "Omission" was the main type of discrepancy found, as in the Tucson study. The researchers concluded that "the location of discrepancies suggests that there are deficiencies in communication between health-care professionals, so future efforts should be directed toward improving interprofessional communication."[113]

Why do adverse events happen?

Some common themes emerge in studies that have focused on adverse events and errors, including the above two studies. Indeed, a whole new field of research has emerged in the past twenty or so years that has explored the basic question of why errors and unintended consequences of events happen. We have probably all heard the phrases "Well, I'm only human" or "No one is perfect" at one time or another. But have you ever thought of why we make mistakes?

Human factors research is an emerging field of research that tries to address these and other related problems. First applied to aviation in an attempt to improve the safety of commercial airlines, it has been more recently applied to health care. Those researchers who try to apply it to health care are often shocked to find so many violations of human factors principles in hospitals. What are these principles? These are essentially key things that should be in place to reduce errors, which include avoiding reliance on memory; simplify, standardize, and improve verbal communication; improve information access; decrease reliance on attention span; and several other principles. The airline industry has attempted to make sure these principles are no longer violated, and as a result, while crashes still happen, aviation safety has dramatically improved in recent years.

Let's take a few minutes to look at one of these principles — *simplify* — and consider how it is often violated in health care. According to the human factors principle *simplify*, each additional step in a process is another opportunity for error. As we have described in this chapter, health care in the hospital setting consists of processes upon processes, some of which have multiple steps, such as getting a medication to a patient. In addition, many of these processes contain multiple handoffs from one individual to another. Each handoff is an opportunity for an error to occur and decreases the likelihood of achieving the intended outcome.

Using an example from the field of aviation, let's imagine that you are going to take a flight from your hometown to Phoenix, Arizona. First, let's assume that you have a direct flight. In that case, there is a pretty good chance that you will arrive in Phoenix on time along with your luggage. Let's now assume that you must make two connections (two handoffs) in order to fly from your hometown to Phoenix and this also includes flying with three different airlines (two other types of handoffs). You may still make it to your destination on time with your luggage, but the likelihood of that happening is far less than with our first hypothetical scenario.

A survey of nurses in one Canadian hospital explored nurses' perceptions of medication safety on their patient care units. In this survey, the nurses felt that the teamwork within the units was excellent. The one area related to adverse drug events and medication process that concerned these nurses the most was handoffs and transitions. Their responses also revealed that several other human factors principles were violated due to inconsistent practices (lack of standardization) and lack of communication. One of the most worrisome results from this study was that only 41% of nurses agreed that their institution had systems in place to ensure that patients were receiving proper medications.[114]

Another way to look at adverse events is to group them into two primary groups. In the first group are *design failures*. This could be where there is a flaw in a process, task, or equipment. For example, if there were a hole in the IV tubing, Bryce would not have received the full dose of his pain medication.

The second group consists of *organizational and environmental failures*. This includes poor education and training (was nurse Stacy properly trained on how to use an IV pump?) or poor team functioning and communication. Also in this group are things such as stress, which can cause health-care teams to function poorly. If one considers many of the most popular medical TV shows over the years, such as *ER* and, more recently, *House*, much of the drama from these shows focuses on dysfunctional health-care teams and members of these teams being forced to make quick decisions under conditions of extreme stress. This makes for interesting TV viewing and also leads to conditions where adverse events are more likely to occur. Indeed, some episodes of these shows have focused on adverse events and errors.

What can be done to reduce and prevent adverse events?
Given this doom and gloom related to adverse events in health care, how can health care be made safer? Clearly, an attempt to follow and adopt human factors principles to health care would be an excellent start, and there are many organizations in Canada that are trying to apply the lessons from this field to health care. For example, a very practical strategy that attempts to help make transitions of care and handoffs related to medication information is called *medication reconciliation*. This phrase essentially means that as patients move across or within health-care settings (for example, from home to the hospital, from hospital to long-term care, from an ICU to a ward, etc.), someone is responsible for ensuring that a complete record of the patient's medications has been obtained. For a patient recently admitted to a hospital, this may mean that a physician, nurse, or pharmacist interviews the patient and calls his or her regular community pharmacy so that a complete and accurate list of the patient's medications can be compiled. In the past few years, medication reconciliation has become a requirement by Accreditation Canada and a core part of our national patient safety initiative, Safer Healthcare Now (www.saferhealthcarenow.ca). During this time, there have been several studies that have also demonstrated the value of this service.[115]

Another strategy to try to improve communication and teamwork among health professionals in the hospital setting that helps to decrease adverse drug events is to add hospital pharmacists to medical rounds. For more information about this, see "The Hospital Pharmacist: An Unsung Hero." Given the present shortage of hospital pharmacists in the country, it remains problematic for many hospitals to include pharmacists on all medical teams as they complete their rounds, but we hope we will see more of this in the next few years.

The Hospital Pharmacist: An Unsung Hero

One of the most effective ways for hospitals to reduce adverse drug events (ADEs) and medication errors and to optimize the drug therapy of their patients is to hire pharmacists and to deploy them on the patient care units, working with other health professionals and joining physicians on medical rounds. For example, one study looked at the impact of adding a pharmacist as a full member of the patient care team in a medical ICU where he participated in medical rounds and in other activities. With the addition of the pharmacist, there was a 66% reduction in preventable ADEs, saving the hospital $270,000 annually.[116] In a study of almost 3 million patients in 885 U.S. hospitals, seven different activities performed by hospital pharmacists were associated with reductions in mortality rate.[117] In a "superstudy" that reviewed the findings of thirty-six other studies, five different hospital pharmacist activities were found to improve outcomes for hospital patients.[118] Finally, authors of another study demonstrated that hospitals gain almost five dollars in benefits for each dollar they spend on hospital pharmacists.[119]

Dr. Jerry Avorn, a well-known physician from New England who has authored many studies about drug use, provided his own personal endorsement in the *Journal of the American Medical Association* ". . . on the important but often unnoticed role of the hospital pharmacist. Few physicians appreciate the quiet yet vital role played by these unassuming colleagues who make it possible for us to propel potions of powerful chemicals through the veins and into the guts of acutely ill inpatients each day, with (all things considered) remarkably few nasty surprises." He added that, "A surgeon who repairs an aortic aneurysm before it ruptures is rightly seen as a hero who saved the patient's life; rarely is similar glory accorded a pharmacist who stops a dose of oxacillin before it reaches a patient with an anaphylaxis-producing penicillin allergy."[120]

So, the next time you are in a hospital, be on the lookout for these heroes in white lab coats.

One study that provided an interesting twist on the question of how to decrease adverse drug events reported on two focus groups of patients and health professionals.[121] In this study, both focus groups were shown trends and examples of medication errors from one hospital. Then a group of health professionals working in that hospital and patients recently discharged from that hospital were asked how the medication-use system might be made safer. The following table contains the responses of both groups. While there was some similarity in the responses of the two groups, most of the responses of the health professionals focused on their own activities while the patients recognized a wider variety of factors.

Top Four Factors Contributing to Medication Errors, as Perceived by Focus Groups of Health Professionals and of Patients[122]

Rank of Factor	As Perceived by Health Professionals	As Perceived by Patients
1	Multitasking	Human error
2	Handwriting	Patients unwilling or unable to provide pertinent information
3	Transcription errors	Overworked doctors and nurses
4	Failure to follow the "5 Rs" (right drug, right dose, right person, right route, right time)	Improper patient identification or failure of patient identification

So you've experienced an error

As Bryce sleeps comfortably in his bed with the new IV pain medication providing relief and comfort, the nursing staff on his unit has their evening shift change. Jan, who takes over for Stacy as the night nurse for Bryce, reviews the nursing medication administration record for Bryce and makes a shocking finding. There is no mark on the record to indicate that Bryce's regularly scheduled pain medication was given in the past twenty-four hours. She checks the nursing administration record, the narcotics sheet, and the patient's medical chart. Perhaps Stacy had simply forgotten to document that she had given Bryce his medication. Or could it be that there was an omission and that somehow the medication was not given to Bryce? As Jan thought more about the situation and reviewed Stacy's notes from the previous shift, she became more concerned. Could this be the reason why Bryce started to feel pain and asked for more pain medication? If this were the case, should the new medication be stopped and the previous medication restarted? If it were indeed an error, should the staff discuss this with Bryce in the morning when he wakes up? Then again, he would never figure it out on his own and perhaps telling him would just cause extra stress. Jan had a lot of issues to discuss with her nursing manager.

Disclosing errors and adverse events in health care is a contentious issue with many different emotions in play, both from the perspective of the health-care professional and the patient. Of course, no health-care professional wants to make an error and feels horrible when one happens. A natural response may be to try to cover it up or deny that it happened at all. See "Hollywood and Disclosing Medical Error" for an example of how this played out in the movie *Ghost Town*.

Hollywood and Disclosing Medical Error

Ghost Town, a Hollywood movie released in 2008, wasn't exactly a blockbuster, but it did provide an interesting perspective on the issue of disclosing error in health care. The lead character, Dr. Pincus, a dentist, has a colonoscopy, and a few days later he suspects something didn't go quite right with the procedure. He returns to the hospital to track down the surgeon who performed the procedure and to find out what really happened.

His surgeon takes him into a small room behind the nursing station, calls in the hospital's physically imposing lawyer, and shuts the door. The ensuing conversation shows what can happen when a hospital tries to hide a serious error.

Dr. Pincus begins the conversation by asking, "Did anything unusual happen during my procedure?" to which the surgeon responds, "Can you please define 'unusual?'"

After the surgeon consults with the hospital's lawyer, Dr. Pincus finds out that he actually died during the colonoscopy for approximately seven minutes before he was revived. The cause was an error with the dosing of the general anesthesia.

Upon finding this out, he then asks, "Where is the anesthesiologist? I want to see him now!"

The surgeon looks quite pleased as she replies, "Oh, he does not work here anymore. You'll be happy to know that here at St. Victor's we have a very strict three-strikes policy."

Dr. Pincus is rightly alarmed at the safety record of his person, asking, "My anesthesiologist had two strikes!?"

His surgeon then tries to settle down the visibly upset Dr. Pincus, requesting, "Okay, let's all calm down, let's just not overdramatize the situation . . . everybody dies."

Dr. Pincus isn't convinced by this excuse, responding, "Yeah, but usually at the end of their life and just the once and forever."

Next, he threatens to sue the hospital, but the lawyer tells him that he can't since he signed a form relieving the medical team and the hospital from any liability related to this health-care error. Dr. Pincus cannot recall signing such a form so the lawyer tells him that he signed it after he passed a post-operative responsiveness test. Even though Dr. Pincus had dotted the "i" in his name with a "love heart," thereby questioning whether he was really in a condition to know what he was signing, the hospital stands by its assertion that legal recourse is not possible and Dr. Pincus will just have to live with the error.[123]

Some have described a culture of fear in health care where, especially in the past, health-care professionals were often fearful of employers and managers who had abrasive or abusive conduct when an error occurred. The health-care professional deemed to be the "cause" of the error would often be made into a scapegoat and would be fired. It is probably not too surprising, then, that many health-care professionals were conflicted about what to do, given that they would essentially be penalized for reporting an error and disclosing it to a patient.

Fortunately, in recent years, there has been an increasing recognition in the health-care community that errors and other adverse events should be disclosed to the patient and these events should be tracked over time and shared outside the hospital setting so that lessons can be shared with other organizations. Hospitals today in Canada have internal systems in place to track all adverse events — sometimes called incidents — such as falls or omissions in care. These systems include mandatory reporting of these events and review of them by both administrators and by a quality improvement or patient safety committee. Hospitals also employ risk managers who look for trends over time and try to implement systems to improve safety. For example, in our scenario, to address whether the nurse forgot to give Bryce his pain medication or simply neglected to document on his medication administration record that the medication was given, there are now electronic medication administration records that will alert the nurse to give the medication.

While hospitals generally have their own policies in place to guide health-care professionals to disclose errors and adverse events with patients, in 2008 the Canadian Patient Safety Institute developed national disclosure guidelines for health-care professionals to use in any setting. The guidelines clearly state that patients have a right to know when such an event occurs. Others have suggested guidelines for disclosing errors that have impacted more than a single patient.[124] In a powerful article in the *New York Times*, one physician shared an error he made and the conflict he faced. As he described in the article: "I knew I had to explain myself, but how much should I say? Like all doctors, I had made errors before, but never one this big — and in my own specialty, too. Should I just tell my patient the facts? Should I apologize?" In the end, he approached the patient and used the "S" word — sorry.[125]

Given the internal systems now in place in hospitals for reporting and disclosing errors and adverse events, more often than not, it will be the health-care professionals who come to the patient to explain what has happened. In many of these cases, as with Bryce, the patient may not have even recognized that something went wrong.

But what should you do if you suspect you've experienced an adverse event? The best approach is to speak to the health-care professionals involved in your care. If you do not feel that your concerns have been taken seriously or that the situation has not been resolved to your satisfaction, you can take your concerns to hospital administrators or to the risk manager. Even if the situation is a misunderstanding and no adverse event actually happened, hospitals who are truly interested in patient safety will, at a minimum, follow up on the complaints of patients and try to figure out whether the concerns are well founded.

You're Being Discharged! Oh Happy Day!

It is finally the day. During medical rounds this morning, Dr. Ryan told Bryce that he is pleased with his progress and the healing of his hip replacement and that Bryce can be discharged back home. There will still be weeks of rehabilitation and an occupational therapist will be visiting Bryce, but at least Bryce is free to return home.

Over the next few hours, Bryce experiences the mad rush of the patient discharge process that is typical of most hospitals. Similar to the admission process, over the next few hours he is seen by untold numbers of health-care professionals, all conveying information and instructions for Bryce and his wife, Pam. It is easy to become overwhelmed by this process, especially when one may be thinking about the joys of home (sleeping in your own bed again, perhaps?) and not completely focused on all the advice these people are providing.

To help minimize both the stress of the discharge process and the challenge in trying to remember what one was told and what one is supposed to do when returning home, we recommend the following actions. First, while verbal instructions are valuable, try to get as much of your discharge advice in a written format that you can later review again from the comfort of your own home. For example, we suggest that you ask for a written list of current medications that you are to take after discharge. Many patients are unsure which medications they have received while in hospital to continue taking and which of the medications that were stopped upon admission should be restarted. It may surprise you that often your community pharmacist is also similarly perplexed unless he or she receives such a list from either the patient or directly from the hospital. So, to prevent your community pharmacist from being forced to become a Sherlock Holmes, this simple piece of information can go a long way in optimizing your care.

Second, for any follow-up activities that are to occur after discharge, be sure that you know who is responsible for coordinating these activities, when they should occur, and to obtain contact information. For example, for the home visits by the occupational therapist, rather than just leaving it that Bryce will be contacted by an occupational therapist sometime in the next few weeks, he should try to clarify the details. If three weeks pass and he still hasn't heard from an occupational therapist, what is he to do?

Third, if your family physician has not been involved in your care while you have been hospitalized, you should ask when your family physician can expect to receive information about your hospitalization from the hospital, the role of your family physician moving forward, and if there is something you should take with you for your family physician. Given that it can take several weeks for a discharge report to reach family physicians in Canada, an unfortunate reality of care in Canada today is that patients sometimes have to step up and act as the intermediary during this care gap.

Conclusion

You are not alone if you find hospitals to be intimidating and mysterious places. You may even be one of many who find it hard just to locate a parking spot when you visit a hospital or you find it a challenge to operate an automated parking meter/machine to pay for parking in a hospital parking lot. And once you enter the walls of a hospital, your anxiety and frustration only continues to mount.

Hopefully we have taken some of this anxiety away as we have described the mysteries of hospitals in this chapter. Yes, hospitals are complex institutions that have their own culture, language, and individuals who engage in seemingly unusual behaviours. And yes, unfortunately, sometimes adverse events do occur in hospitals. However, at the core of these buildings, one will find some of the most caring and compassionate individuals on the planet. Hospitals are indeed modern-day cathedrals in which miracles happen daily.

CHAPTER NINE

HOME
SWEET HOME

The Heart of Medication Management

Now that we have completed our tour of several health-care settings — the physician's office, the pharmacy, the emergency department, and the hospital — we return to where we began: your home. In this chapter, we will explore many issues related to medication use in the home, such as creating your own personal health-care centre, the role of ongoing monitoring for side effects, and the emerging use of personal health records. First, though, we will address what is perhaps the most challenging aspect of medication use in the home — medication adherence. We'll explore this issue in-depth, discussing why it is such a challenge for so many Canadians and providing some tips and advice on how to remember to take your medications.

Do I Really Have to Take This Stuff?

Erica is back in her bathroom, trying to clean the spots out of another blouse. She has lost track of how many battles she has had with her four-year-old daughter, Bianca, trying to get the liquid antibiotic into her mouth. Most of the episodes end up like this one — five minutes of her daughter's screaming and most of the medication ending up on her blouse and on the kitchen floor. This daily battle has been going on three times a day for seven days now. The doctor wrote the prescription for a ten-day supply of the sticky liquid, and her pharmacist reminded Erica to give it to Bianca until the medication was completely gone. However, Bianca's strep throat seems all better now and she is back to her usual feisty self. Does Erica really need to engage in this battle of the wills for another three days?

Peter has been taking a new prescription for high blood pressure for about a month now. His doctor told him that he had reached a point in his life where medication was needed as changes to his diet and additional exercise over the past year have not been enough to lower his blood pressure to a normal level. His doctor told him that taking this medication would help lower his blood pressure and prevent more serious complications in the future. However, Peter feels worse than ever and he can't imagine having to take this medication for the rest of his life. Perhaps he could just cut back on the medication and take half a tablet and not tell anyone? Technically, he'd still be taking his medication and perhaps the side effects would go away?

Shirley takes a big, heavy sigh, resting back in her favourite easy chair, home from a trip to her doctor and pharmacy. It has not been a good day. Her doctor shared with her the results from her latest bone density test, which indicated that she needs to start a new drug to treat her osteoporosis. Her doctor wrote a prescription that Shirley took to her community pharmacy to have filled. At the pharmacy, her pharmacist told her that her senior's drug plan did not cover that medication, proceeded to tell her how much it would cost, and said he could call Shirley's physician to see about getting the medication changed to a less expensive one. Shirley was embarrassed by this whole situation and she asked the pharmacist for the prescription back and came home, trying to decide whether she should have it filled. If she cut back on her grocery budget or made fewer trips to see her son, she might just be able to go back to a pharmacy (a different one, of course, where she could put this embarrassing moment behind her) and get the prescription filled. Or she could opt for the less expensive medication — but did that mean it would be less effective as well?

These three scenarios all address the same issue — medication adherence. If you have ever been in a similar situation as the individuals in these scenarios or have asked the question "Do I really have to take this stuff?" you are not alone. Even the British singer Morrissey included the following as lyrics in one of his more recent songs: "Diazepam (that's Valium), temazepam . . . lithium . . . How long must I stay on this stuff?"[126]

How prevalent is the issue of poor or non-adherence? It is notoriously tricky for health-care researchers to answer that question as it is a very complex problem. Some patients may avoid going to see a doctor altogether because they are worried about being diagnosed with a condition and do not want to start taking a new medication. Other patients will leave the doctor's office with a prescription in hand and never go to a pharmacy to have it filled. Others will drop off the prescription at a pharmacy to have it filled but never pick up the filled prescription. And still others will pick up their prescription from the pharmacy but once at home won't take it as directed. Any accurate measure of non-adherence should capture the problem at all these different stages of the medication-use system.

While estimates of the magnitude of non-adherence are difficult to measure due to its complex nature, both physicians and the general public admit it is a considerable problem. As we reviewed in "International Comparisons on Prescription Access, Affordability, Quality, and Safety" on page 23, 24% of Canadian primary care physicians believe that their patients *often* experience difficulty paying for prescriptions while 18% of adults with chronic conditions admitted they do not fill a prescription or skip doses due to costs.

This leads us to the next issue — what exactly is adherence? Certainly, even among health-care researchers and clinicians a variety of terms are used, such as *compliance, concordance, persistence,* and *adherence.* We prefer the term *intelligent adherence.* According to this term, the patient or caregiver should consent to the goals (therapeutic objectives) of the medication, know the signs of therapeutic success and side effects, know when to expect side effects, and know what to do if they appear. This is much more beneficial to the patient than simply continuing to take a medication as directed by the physician even if side effects appear or if the medication doesn't appear to be working. Most importantly, then, the term *intelligent adherence* suggests an active role for the patient that includes responsibilities.

Using the term *intelligent adherence*, each of the three scenarios we introduced in this chapter could have been constructively resolved. In Erica and Bianca's example, if the antibiotic suspension was so unpalatable to Bianca, Erica could have easily called the pharmacist and discovered that some antibiotics come in a variety of different flavours. In certain cases, the pharmacist may be able to specially prepare a suspension just for unique tastes (peaches and cream for Bianca, perhaps?).

In Paul's example, if the medication for high blood pressure was causing a side effect, Paul could have made an appointment to talk to his physician about this rather than secretively cutting back on the dosage. In doing this, Paul's physician would have shared with him that there are several different options for drug therapy for high blood pressure and she might have prescribed a different medication. However, this step may not even have been necessary as certain side effects subside after a short period of time. Also, the dosage may have just simply been too high and could have been reduced — but *only* with the physician's knowledge and active monitoring, not independently as Paul was considering. If Paul had proceeded with his initial course of action, there is a good chance that at his next visit with his doctor, she would question why Paul's blood pressure hadn't lowered despite his starting this new drug and she may have even ended up increasing the dosage.

Finally, in Shirley's example, it may be true that her drug plan didn't pay for the medication that had been prescribed. However, in many cases, if her physician completed a special form or made an appeal to the drug plan as to why it should be covered (perhaps Shirley had tried other drugs and they hadn't helped with her osteoporosis or Shirley was allergic to other options), it may have been covered. Thus, a patient who engages in intelligent adherence and works with his or her health professionals is more likely to achieve an optimal outcome from prescription drugs.

As our three scenarios also illustrate, there are many different causes of non-adherence. The following table outlines seventeen different characteristics that are known to have a relationship to adherence. For many patients, several of the seventeen characteristics may apply to their situation so it is not surprising that so many Canadians struggle with this issue. In fact, as is shown in "Intelligent Adherence and Placebos" (page 223), even different types of placebo drugs can impact adherence in different ways.

Characteristics Related to Medication-Taking Behaviour[127]

Characteristic	Direction of Findings
Treatment regimen characteristics	
Dosing frequency	The greater the frequency (number of times a day a medication is prescribed to be taken), the greater the non-adherence.
Medication side effects	The worse the actual or perceived side effects, the greater the non-adherence.
Medication costs	Even for those with insurance, the higher the cost (in dollars), the greater the non-adherence.
Patient sociodemographic characteristics	
Age	Younger patients are generally less adherent than older patients. However, as patients age and begin to lose memory, they sometimes forget to take their medication.

Characteristic	Direction of Findings
Patient sociodemographic characteristics	
Gender	Men are generally, but not always, less adherent than women.
Socioeconomic status (SES)	The lower the SES, particularly as related to low education, the greater the non-adherence.
Patient psychological characteristics	
Personality characteristics	No clear, unequivocal trends have emerged, but hostility might be predictive of non-adherence, and conscientiousness might predict adherence.
Strong belief that taking the medication will help one to reach certain goals (high self-efficacy)	The higher the self-efficacy for taking one's medicine, the greater the adherence.
Patient depression	Only among the most severely depressed patients is there a relationship with non-adherence.
Social support and social environment	
Satisfaction with, and quality of, support	Generally, the more satisfied the patient is with the quality of support perceived (or received from friends and family), the greater the adherence.
Size of social network	No clear association with adherence.
Family environment	More cohesion and less conflict in the family are associated with greater adherence.

Physician and physician practice style characteristics	
Effective communication to and from	If the physician engages in this type of the patient and physician communication, there is greater adherence.
Mutual trust	If either the patient or the physician distrusts the other, adherence will suffer.
Willingness to answer the patient's questions	The more the physician is willing to answer questions and provide information, the greater the patient satisfaction, but this has no effect on adherence.
Number of patients seen by the physician in a given period of time	Paradoxically, medication adherence is greater among patients whose physicians see more patients per week.
Physician job satisfaction	Satisfied physicians have more adherent patients.

Intelligent Adherence and Placebos

While one could easily see why two different drugs that cause different side effects might impact adherence differently, you may be surprised that different placebos can also impact adherence differently. Author Daniel E. Moerman explores this interesting phenomenon in his book *Meaning, Medicine and the "Placebo Effect."* He reviews how "brand-name" placebos can work better than "generic" placebos and that placebos can differ in their effectiveness greatly across different countries. For example, in one of the more bizarre findings in his book, blue placebos are better sedatives than red ones with the exception being in Italian men, in whom red placebos work better.

He also concludes that patients who are more adherent with their placebo drugs do better than patients who are less adherent. So, intelligent adherence seems to matter even with placebos![128]

Given that adherence is a complex problem that is impacted by many different factors, how then can adherence be improved? The following table contains many different factors that patients are advised to consider when working with researchers and clinicians to improve adherence.

What Successful Adherence Strategies Look Like[129]

Medication adherence can improve when . . .
your health-care provider appraises your unique needs.
your health intervention is pegged to your level of health literacy.
contact between you and your health professionals (e.g., physicians, pharmacists, etc.) is increased.
you are included in problem-solving tasks (e.g., how to ensure that adherence doesn't suffer while you are on vacation).
you are educated to recognize beliefs about adherence that may be incorrect (e.g., you will become addicted to a medication [if not a narcotic, as these are, in fact, habit forming]).
your health-care professionals work with you to let you know that adherence will be evaluated, with repeated and explicit monitoring by health professionals.
you are encouraged to have positive expectations about improvements in adherence.
you are engaged in behaviour that stresses the importance of adherence.
you make an explicit commitment, either in writing or verbally, to take the medication as prescribed.
you receive encouragement and social support from other patients, friends, and/or family members.
you receive some form of reinforcement for successful adherence.

Strategies for improving adherence can be grouped into several different categories. First, there are strategies to help you organize your medications. These can be simple adherence aids, dosettes, or pillboxes in which you can place a day's or week's supply of medications and which can be purchased at most pharmacies. Some of the more complex pillboxes have up to twenty-eight different slots (four slots a day for each of the seven days of the week). In a more advanced version of this, many pharmacies will do this work for you for an extra fee, placing your medications into individual "bubbles" in a sheet with a foil backing, typically called a blister pack. Many residents of long-term care facilities receive their medications in this fashion, which can be very helpful for patients taking several medications or who get easily confused about when to take each medication. Some patients find that writing their medication schedule on a calendar is helpful too, and they cross off the corresponding calendar item each time they take a medication.

A survey of 135 independently living middle-aged and senior adults in New Brunswick provides some insights into how often these types of adherence aids are used and the perceived value of them by the adults who use them. In these adults, almost one out of four used a pillbox for all medications, while many others used some sort of combination of a pillbox, prescription vials, and blister packs. Only 18.5% used no adherence aid at all. The patients who used a pillbox reported that they found it useful for remembering time and day of dosage and useful for remembering the correct amount, believed that it was effective in helping them to take medications correctly, and felt there has been an improvement in their adherence once they started using it. [130] Not bad results for an inexpensive little piece of plastic! If you are taking several medications, we certainly recommend that you purchase and use a pillbox. As the New Brunswick survey shows, pillboxes are not only for seniors. If you purchase one at a pharmacy and ask, a pharmacist will show you how to load it for the first time for free.

A second type of strategy deals with reminders to take medications. Some patients may be lucky enough to have a relative willing to call them each time they need to take a medication, but these types of relatives are hard to find indeed. Some may have their e-mail or scheduler program on their computer remind them with alerts or receive a reminder from their iPhone or BlackBerry. Some individuals have difficulty remembering to have refills of their prescription filled on time. This can be especially problematic if they run out of the medication on a holiday weekend when pharmacies and physician offices are closed or have reduced hours. Many pharmacies now offer automated telephone reminder calls for free, whereby the patient will receive a call a couple of days before the prescription is due to be refilled. Some pharmacies take this a step further and have programs in which patients can enrol for free to have their prescription automatically refilled at the pharmacy. If these types of programs may be of interest to you, we suggest you speak to your pharmacist about how to enrol.

A third type of strategy deals with increasing the patient's knowledge or understanding of the medication and what the consequences could be if the medication were to be stopped abruptly. As you saw in the previous table, many of the most effective strategies for improving adherence centre around this type of strategy. It is clear that if patients are unsure of how a medication is helping them, are unclear about its purpose, or are unsure what to do if side effects appear, they are at a greater risk of being non-adherent. In an intelligent adherence approach, the patient is clear on all these points and actively works with his or her health-care team to monitor whether the medication is meeting its intended purpose.

The most effective approach to improving adherence is when a combination of three of the above strategies is used, built around the unique needs of the patient.

A Health-Care Centre in Your Home?

In this section we would like to provide some practical advice for medication use in your home, whether you live in a 5,000-square-foot McMansion or a small studio apartment. While we do not recommend that your home become the next regional hospital in your area, we do suggest that you have a small "health-care centre" in your place of residence where all of your health-care related documents, information, medications, and other supplies are located. For many of you, this may be a cabinet that is out of the reach of children in your kitchen or pantry. For others, this may be in a home office or bedroom. We will not dictate where we feel this health-care centre must be located, but we do have some general advice following this easy to remember acronym: CARE.

C is for comprehensive. Your health-care centre should be comprehensive, meaning that it should be more than a small shelf with a few prescriptions and over-the-counter medications. A comprehensive centre will contain the following items in addition to your medications (and the dosette you will soon purchase, as per our suggestion a few minutes ago). First, the phone numbers of your physicians, pharmacy, other allied health professionals such as occupational therapist and physiotherapist, regional poison centre, and provincial health-care triage number (if applicable). Make sure these are easy to find — you don't want to be searching for the regional poison centre number when you suspect your toddler has downed the ice melter pellets. Second, you should have copies of all your health insurance information — a copy of your provincial or territorial health card, your private health insurance information, and so on. Third, create a list of all your medications, including dosage and purpose, and any allergies you might have. It is important to have this information on your person in a wallet or purse, but an extra copy should also be kept in your centre. A common problem with these lists is that they are out of date so be sure to update it each time your medications change. Fourth, this is a great place to keep a family first-aid kit. And lastly, be sure to include a copy of *Take as Directed* (okay, we couldn't resist).

A is for accessible. You should make your centre accessible and inaccessible at the same time. Allow us to explain. Your centre should be accessible to you and in a place where you'll remember to take your medications and where you'll easily find a number in case of an emergency. However, it should also be in a place where it is hard for children to access the contents inside your centre. Even if you are a grandparent or don't have children living in your place of residency, consider the times you may have children visiting. To a three-year-old, the pills that Papa or Grandma are taking look a lot like candy. Also, if you have a cat or dog, you'll want to make sure that medications are far away from them. One of us (NM) has an Airedale terrier, Winnie, as a family pet, who has devoured all sorts of food and substances, including wire scouring pads, without any apparent ill effect, but this is definitely the exception to the rule for animals. You may also be living with a person who has dementia or a desire to self-harm, and you will want to make sure this person does not access and take your medications. Perhaps if this is your reality, you need to consider having your medications in a locked box or drawer.

R is for remove. It is amazing how quickly bottles of various medications can build up over time. When you change the batteries in your smoke detector, remember to spend an extra few minutes by going through your health-care centre, reviewing the expiration dates of old medications, both prescription and over-the-counter products. If you do find expired medications, rather than damaging the environment by throwing them into the garbage or dumping the contents down the sink, take them to your pharmacy for free disposal. They will be incinerated at a remote location along with other expired medications.

E is for extreme environments. The enemies of most medications are moisture and temperature extremes. Some medications do require refrigeration; however, your pharmacist should tell you this at the pharmacy, along with placing a sticker on the medication, if this applies to your medication. Unless extremely well ventilated, bathrooms are not an ideal place for medications due to the high moisture content in these rooms. Most of us do not have humidors that control moisture perfectly, but we all have areas in our place of residence in which medications are less susceptible to extremes of moisture and/or temperature. Remember that medications should not be kept in cars due to temperature extremes, especially in our harsh Canadian climate.

The Patient's Role in Between Doctor and Pharmacy Visits

As you might suspect from the title of the chapter, the home is the key place for medication management for most Canadians. Yes, there will be many Canadians who will visit our country's emergency departments or who will be admitted to a hospital this year. Others may even spend a majority of the year in a long-term care facility. Nevertheless, for most Canadians, a large percentage of their 365 days this year will be spent outside these settings, either managing their medications at home or elsewhere on vacation or on business. While intelligent adherence and CARE are important concepts to remember, the key reason why the home is the heart for medication management is the patient's role in active, ongoing monitoring.

What is meant by the concept of monitoring? It certainly has a lot of different meanings, depending on the context. For an automobile, it may refer to short-term tasks such as making sure there is gas in the tank and medium- and long-term checks such as ensuring that the tire pressure is okay and that the car is being serviced regularly. Regarding medications, monitoring means watching for side effects and whether the goal of the medication is being met. It also means the detection and resolution of problems before they become more serious adverse drug events. In addition, there may be other key activities that assist with these things. For a patient with diabetes, this could include daily monitoring of blood glucose levels and long-term monitoring of annual foot and eye examinations and measuring diabetic glucose ("sugar") control over an extended period of time via glycosylated hemoglobin (hemoglobin A1C). Many other medications require regular lab tests to assess the amount of the medication in the body itself, such as medications for thyroid conditions. Other medications require ongoing monitoring of potential side effects, such as liver damage with some medications for cholesterol. For monitoring to work best, it needs to be a collaborative effort between the patient and his or her health-care team.

How important is ongoing monitoring? In one study, three panels of physicians that included family physicians, geriatricians, and clinical pharmacologists were asked how different types of adverse drug events could best be prevented in seniors. The physicians could choose from eight different strategies in any combination. Which strategy was most frequently chosen? Monitoring.[131] Other researchers have argued that monitoring "may be the most promising way to improve medication use."[132]

Another study of more than 22,000 seniors in Halifax, Nova Scotia, also demonstrates the importance of monitoring and what can happen when it is not done. In this study, seniors were followed to see whether they had an emergency department visit or hospitalization that was drug-related and preventable. Over the course of the two-year study, roughly one in every nine seniors experienced one or more of these events. Several of the most commonly occurring events seemed to result when patients fell through the cracks of the health-care system and where ongoing monitoring was forgotten or omitted. For example, there were 519 seniors in the study who were on a drug for a thyroid condition. Guidelines at the time of the study recommended that regular laboratory testing be done to determine whether the drug was being dosed appropriately. In these seniors, the test was not done for some reason and they all had an emergency department visit or were hospitalized due to hyperthyroidism as a result.[133] These visits and admissions could all have been prevented if regular monitoring was done.

So, what can you do to ensure that ongoing monitoring is done? When you are prescribed a new drug by your physician, ask him or her which side effects to watch for, when they might occur, and what you should do if you experience them. You should also ask if there is any daily monitoring that should be done, as with many drugs for asthma and diabetes, or any long-term monitoring that needs to be done, as with some drugs for cholesterol and others. By being an informed and active participant in your own care, you are more likely to achieve an optimal outcome from your medications.

The Future at Your Fingertips?

For most Canadians, the amount of information they actually have about their own conditions, medications, diagnoses, laboratory tests, procedures, and other health-care experiences is typically very low. Some may keep a list of medications, as we have suggested, and others may have done some research at a library or on the internet about a condition they have, but for most Canadians that is the extent of it. A receptionist at a physician's office may call to say that the lab test result came back and it was normal, but that is usually the end of the discussion. We may see the physician making notes during a visit or a nurse writing in a chart beside a hospital bed, but we are never privy to what is being written. Even if asked at that moment what they have just written, many health professionals may be hesitant to share the content of their note. Consider the following scenario.

Leanne pours a cup of herbal tea and sits down at the computer in her home office, logging on to a website to access her personal health record. Earlier in the day, she had visited her family doctor, who prescribed a new medication for her migraines, and she had the prescription filled at her neighbourhood pharmacy. Both her physician and pharmacist were helpful and told her how this new medication works, when to take it, and what side effects to watch for. Despite the great information they shared, Leanne didn't really take it all in due to the lingering pain from last night's migraine attack and the hustle and bustle of the physician's office and pharmacy. She is hoping to really grasp it all here in the comfort of her home with the help of her personal health record.

Leanne accesses her entire medical history, including all the information from her last migraine attack–related emergency department visit one month ago. Through a secure link, her hospital has allowed her to import her complete record from this visit, including all lab tests done and drugs administered. She also scans her complete prescription profile history, provided electronically by her local pharmacy. She notes the latest entry for the new prescription that she just picked up an hour ago, and she uses the software on the website to check for interactions with the other medications she is taking, plus reads up some more on this new medication. After spending a few minutes reading, she is concerned about a side effect from this medication that she doesn't remember her pharmacist or physician mentioning and emails her physician's receptionist to make an appointment. With her current prescription profile updated with this new medication, before logging off the website, she prints off two wallet-sized versions of her updated medication record, one for her purse and one for her home health-care centre.

This scenario is based on the existing capabilities of personal health record services such as Dossia, Google Health, Indivo, and Microsoft's HealthVault, which are freely available today. Most of the functions that Leanne used, such as accessing records from hospitals and pharmacies, are only limited to a small number of partnering health-care organizations in the United States at the time of writing this book but are expected to increase over time both within and outside the United States. In Canada, a pilot project incorporating some aspects of the above scenario was completed with more than 500 patients with diabetes and published in the *Canadian Medical Association Journal* in 2009. In this study, the electronic medical records from the patients' family physicians were linked to an internet-based tool where patients could view and track their laboratory tests and other measures of their diabetes control. By the end of the study, patients who experienced this intervention improved clinically and were satisfied with their care.[134] Still, we are quite far off from making this an everyday scenario in Canada today.

Certainly, issues concerning privacy, patient confidentiality, and information access that need to be fully explored. Still, health-care information — so vital to patients who are fully engaged participants in their care and who are actively helping monitor the outcomes from their medications — is sorely lacking for patients in their homes. It will be interesting to watch the evolution of personal health records in the coming years.

Conclusion

Most Canadians will begin their prescription or non-prescription drug therapy at a physician's office, a pharmacy, an emergency department, or a hospital. While the beginning steps of the medication-use system are critical — receiving the right diagnosis, receiving the right drug and dosage, receiving the right information about the drug, and having an opportunity to ask questions — it is medication use at home that often determines whether the goals of medication will be achieved in a given patient. As we have reviewed, the concepts of intelligent adherence, a home health-care centre, and ongoing monitoring are critical. Typically, however, our health-care system places little emphasis on the role of medication management in the home. We hope that after reading this chapter, you'll agree with us that the home is the heart of medication management.

CHAPTER TEN

DEMYSTIFYING DRUG AND HEALTH-CARE INFORMATION

The Search for Reliable Reading

Now that we have completed our tour of the health-care system, let's turn to the issue of where to find trustworthy information about medications, diseases, and other health-care-related issues. Many of you are probably wondering, "Where do I turn to learn more about the drugs I take?"

Before we tackle this issue, however, we are going to take a step back and review how new drugs come to market through clinical trials and how the scientific literature is generated. We suspect most of you will not be interested in deciphering the original scientific studies published in health-care journals. Nevertheless, all information about drugs — whether from a newspaper or magazine article, a website, or some other source — is ultimately based on these published studies. Thus, an understanding of how drugs are developed and how new scientific literature is published is key in helping to choose trustworthy drug information sources.

We will also spend some time discussing that big blue book that physicians and pharmacists frequently flip through to find out more information about drugs and the written information you may receive from your pharmacist. Finally, we'll provide our recommendations for reputable websites for drug information and health care in general.

The Journey from Drug Discovery to Bedside and Beyond

The process from developing a new drug to the drug being used in everyday medical practice — sometimes called *drug discovery to bedside* — is a long one fraught with many challenges. As the pharmaceutical industry asserts, the journey can easily take a decade or longer and cost hundreds of millions of dollars, although the exact cost is difficult to determine. In addition, success, defined by a new drug coming to the market and being used by the medical community, is not guaranteed. Again, precise success rates are difficult to determine, but the odds aren't good: several drugs fail to complete the journey for each drug that does. It is true that pharmaceutical companies typically generate large corporate profits and patients and other payers are justified in their concern about high drug costs, but we do need to acknowledge the great expense and high risk of the drug development process. Moreover, as a society, we place value on the development of new drug products that cure or prevent disease or reduce the signs and symptoms of disease. Regardless of one's stance on the pharmaceutical industry, it is safe to say that all Canadians would prefer a world in which pharmaceutical companies are successful in developing innovative drug products that improve the quality of our citizens' lives.

Let's take a closer look at the journey that a drug product takes from discovery to bedside and beyond. The process typically starts with the selection of chemical compounds that are thought to have an impact within the human body. This research may occur within a pharmaceutical company, a biotechnology company, or in a university laboratory. Sometimes these chemical compounds might be slight variations of an existing drug, with the hope of improving the side-effect profile or the effectiveness of the existing drug.

Once the compound is thought to demonstrate promise and a patent has been obtained, the clinical trial process begins. Three phases of clinical trials (usually noted by the Roman numerals I, II, and III) are typically completed before a drug comes to market, with a fourth phase after a drug is marketed. In phase I trials, the focus is testing the safety of the drug, which is usually done with a small group of patients (typically under 100). In phase II trials, there are further evaluations of safety, although the focus shifts to potential benefits and the impact the drug may have on a disease or condition. This phase is also completed on a relatively small group of patients (usually 300 or less). In phase III trials, a larger number of patients is included (sometimes up to tens of thousands of patients) to gather more information about the benefits of the drug, its safety profile, and often to compare the new drug to existing therapies. For some drugs used to treat very rare conditions, though, a phase III trial may include 100 patients or less.

The goal of the clinical trial process is to determine the side-effect profile of the drug, its optimal dosing and dosage forms (tablet, capsule, solutions, injection, inhalation, etc.), and, of course, how well it works in the patients who have the condition for which it is being tested. This last characteristic of a drug is called *efficacy*. Later in this section, we'll review the important difference between efficacy and effectiveness — how the drug works in the real world. If you are interested in finding out more about clinical trials that are currently active, see "The One-Stop Shop for Clinical Trials."

The One-Stop Shop for Clinical Trials

You may have wondered whether there are any promising new drugs being tested for a disease such as type II diabetes, prostate cancer, or multiple sclerosis. To track clinical trials, you can visit www.clinical-trials.gov, which was set up by the U.S. government a few years ago and is maintained by the U.S. National Institutes of Health. At the time of writing this chapter, there were more than 83,000 trials in the database from 171 countries. The website contains a search engine so you can look for trials for specific conditions in specific geographical areas. Once you find a trial, you can learn about its status (not yet recruiting, recruiting, completed, etc.), its purpose, which patients are eligible to enrol in the study, and contact information if you are interested in enrolling in the trial. In addition to this detailed information about each clinical trial, the website also contains many areas of special interest, such as sections that explain all about clinical trials and provide information on recently published trials. Companies completing at least part of their clinical trial in the United States are required by law to include their information on this website so you can be sure it is fairly comprehensive.

If the company holding the patent of the drug believes that the drug product would be worth bringing to market, it must then apply to the appropriate regulatory agency in each country in order to allow prescribing of the drug. In Canada, this agency is Health Canada. Typically, Health Canada reviews details of the phase III clinical trials, and if it determines that the drug is both safe and efficacious, it will grant a Notice of Compliance (NOC). At that point, the drug can be legally prescribed in Canada. In some cases, for diseases in which there is an urgent need for improved drug therapy, such as for cancer and HIV/AIDS, Health Canada will grant a Notice of Compliance with conditions (NOC/c), but in such instances the pharmaceutical company must agree to provide additional information once the clinical trials have been completed. One additional step in Canada for brand name drugs is that the drugs must be reviewed by the Patented Medicines Prices Review Board (www.pmprb-cepmb.gc.ca) to set the maximum pricing of the drug. The price is based on the average price in several other western, industrialized nations and whether the drug is deemed to be a "breakthrough" product.

As we reviewed in Chapters 2 and 3, just because a drug can be legally prescribed in Canada doesn't mean that it will be widely prescribed. Since the majority of Canadians have drug insurance either through a public drug plan or a private drug plan, pharmaceutical companies submit additional documentation to these insurers in an attempt to have their drugs covered, or listed, on their formularies. Once a drug has been listed on a formulary, pharmaceutical companies will send sales representatives to visit physicians and pharmacists in an attempt to educate them about the new drug product. The company also has the exclusive right to manufacture and sell that drug until its patent runs out, after which other companies can apply through Health Canada to manufacture the product. These other companies produce versions of the drug, which are called *generics*. Generics have the same active drug and may or may not look nearly identical to the original brand name product. Generic drugs typically are priced at 60% to 80% of the price of the brand name products. Complicating this further, some pharmaceutical companies also produce their own generic versions of their brand name products after the initial patent runs out, in an attempt to keep market share.

It is important to note that a company must go through each of the above steps (starting with phase I clinical trials) for each different use, or indication, of the drug. For example, when Health Canada grants its Notice of Compliance, it is only for a specific indication. Many drugs on the market today can be used for multiple health conditions and thus have gone through this process many times. Sometimes the brand name of the same drug compound may be different for different health conditions. For example, the drug minoxidil is sold as Loniten for high blood pressure and sold as Rogaine for hair regrowth.

The last phase of clinical trials (phase IV, or post-marketing surveillance) occurs after a drug product comes to market. In this phase, the drug is being tested for *effectiveness* — its performance in the real world in patients with multiple conditions and in patients who did not fit the profile of patients in the controlled clinical trials. This phase has become recognized in recent years as being extremely important as drugs do not always have the same side-effect profile when they are widely prescribed. Interestingly, efficacy and effectiveness can differ considerably. There have been some notable examples (the anti-inflammatory Vioxx, hormone replacement therapy to treat symptoms of menopause, and others) where, once used widely, concerns arose about the drugs that were not evident in the clinical trials. As we note in the final chapter, a new initiative in our country, the Drug Safety and Effectiveness Network, has been established and has received $32 million from the federal government over its first five years to better monitor the performance of drugs in the real world.

A Guide to the Scientific Literature

Now that we have reviewed the drug development process, let's explore how information about this process makes it into the scientific literature.

As phase II and III clinical trials of drugs are completed, the researchers and authors of those studies will typically present their findings at scientific and health-care meetings to clinicians and other researchers. The results may be presented verbally (a podium presentation) or in a graphical format called a research poster. Typically, a short written summary of the presentation consisting of 250 to 500 words, called a *research abstract*, is prepared and published by the conference organizers in conjunction with a podium or poster presentation. Often, the initial reports carried in the media about a promising new drug come from these research abstracts at scientific meetings.

The next step is the publication of the full study results in a scientific and/or health-care journal. It may take six months to eighteen months from the time a study is completed until it is published in such a journal. These articles are usually at least 2,500 words in length and go into far more depth than the research presented at scientific meetings. Why does the process of publishing the full results take so long? Scientific journals in all fields use a process called peer-review, whereby "peers" (experts in the field who did not participate in the study) are asked to rigorously assess the research methods used in the study, the analysis of the results, and the conclusions made by the researchers. While the process usually serves the research community well, there are exceptions and limitations, as noted in "When Peer Review Goes Amiss."

When Peer Review Goes Amiss

In fall 2009, one of the major news stories worldwide was the so-called "climategate" scandal. Some computer hackers retrieved emails from a climate change research centre in England and made the messages public. The emails suggested that the researchers were engaged in unethical behaviours to repress the findings of colleagues in their field who had opposing viewpoints. (Of course, there is the question of the unethical behaviour of hacking computers, but that is another issue . . .) Many of these behaviours dealt with the peer review process, such as searching for reasons why these opposing research papers were flawed. Here's a sample from one of the hacked emails: "I got a paper to review . . . If published as is, this paper could really do some damage . . . It won't be easy to dismiss out of hand as the math appears to be correct theoretically (. . .) I am really sorry but I have to nag about that review — Confidentially I now need a hard and if required, extensive case for rejecting."[135]

Regardless of your perspective on climate change, the public release of these emails certainly raised questions about, and harmed the message of, these researchers. We may rightly ask, "If the peer review process for climate change researchers went amiss, could this happen in other fields too?" The quick answer to that question is "yes." While this type of evidence of tampering with the peer review process may not exist in all other fields, certainly the opportunity for it exists. Most journal editors ask their reviewers to assess scientific papers along strict criteria and ask three, four, or even more individuals to review each paper in an attempt to minimize subjectivity and bias. However, in some areas of research, including research for some diseases or drugs, there may be a very limited pool of suitable researchers from which to draw reviewers. Also, while the names of the researchers who authored the paper being reviewed are typically blinded to the reviewers, often it does not take too much work on the part of the reviewers to figure out who wrote the paper, and if there is a personal bias against an individual, this may bear out in the review. Alas, the peer review process employed by the scientific community is a human one, and as we have reviewed elsewhere in this book, to err is human. We will likely continue to rely on the peer review process, while being alert for abuses of the process in all fields, including in the clinical trials of drugs.

Another important barometer of the quality of any scientific paper is the quality of the journal in which the paper is published. Those who frequently watch TV for the latest news about new drugs, surgical techniques, or lifestyle activities such as exercise and diet and their impact on health likely recall hearing the names of some of the more prominent health-care journals. These include the *New England Journal of Medicine*, the *Journal of the American Medical Association (JAMA)*, the *British Medical Journal (BMJ)*, and, in Canada, the *Canadian Medical Association Journal (CMAJ)*. What makes these journals so special? These and a few other select health-care journals are known by researchers as being top-tiered journals. This means that they are well respected, articles published in these journals tend to garner considerable media attention, and, what is important to the scientific community, they have a high citation index. The citation index, or impact factor, refers to the number of times a given study is referenced, or cited, by other studies. A citation index is not a perfect indicator of the quality of a journal, but it does give an important perspective. Often, if a researcher submits a paper to one of these top-tiered journals and the journal declines to publish it, the researcher will then submit the paper to a journal in the next tier of journals and so on, until the paper is accepted for publication.

Finally, another consideration when assessing the quality of a scientific study is the funding source and the financial disclosures of the researchers who participated in the study. As you might expect, if a study is funded by the company whose product is being evaluated, it does raise suspicion about the study itself, whether that product is a new dishwasher, car, or drug. This is one reason why resources such as *Consumer Reports* are so valuable, as at least theoretically, an evaluation by an independent third party is less biased. In Canada, much health-care research is funded by the Canadian Institutes of Health Research, which uses a peer review process to award grants. However, most clinical trials of new drugs, both here in Canada and worldwide, are funded by the pharmaceutical industry. This does not mean that the results of studies should be automatically dismissed out of hand, but it is an important point to keep in mind. Due to the large cost of conducting clinical trials, it is hard to imagine the funding source of these studies changing in the foreseeable future.

"Wait a Minute . . . Now *That* Is Bad for Me?"

Joanne shuts off the TV, shaking her head, and turns to her husband, who is doing a crossword puzzle in the chair next to her. "Can you believe that news?" she asks without waiting for a response from him. "Now there is a new study saying that the drug I have been taking for ten years causes some bad reactions and doctors should be leery when prescribing it. What am I supposed to do? Stop taking it? I thought this drug was supposed to be helping me. I don't know what to believe anymore!"

Most of us have been in a similar situation where we have heard conflicting information about the benefits or harm of something we eat, a drug we take, or something else we do. While we are told alcohol is addictive and destroys our livers and chocolate makes us fat, we've likely also seen studies that support the antioxidant properties of red wine and dark chocolate. Like Joanne, it is sometimes difficult to know what to believe and how to react. Some people may be tempted to give up listening to the news at all and may question whether scientists and researchers just come up with these studies to confuse us all!

In many cases, there are good reasons for what may actually be, in fact, conflicting results. As we have reviewed, often there is a difference between the efficacy of a drug in the controlled environment of a clinical trial and the effectiveness of a drug in the real world. In other cases, perhaps the initial findings were based on small studies whereas it took time for a larger, long-term study to be completed and to yield more information. It is also important to note that the change isn't always in a bad direction. That is, often new potential uses and benefits of existing drugs are found over time in subsequent studies.

Still, we are left with the reality that there may be multiple studies of the same drug that yield conflicting results. So, what can be done to help reduce potential confusion? Certainly, there are some tools being used by clinicians and researchers alike to try to sift through conflicting data and to then pass on this information in a meaningful way to patients. Researchers are increasingly relying on "super-studies" called *meta analyses* and *systematic reviews* that help to compile the results of multiple studies and to make sense of it all. For example, there may be ten studies, six of which suggest that Drug X prevents strokes and four of which say it does not. Rather than simply saying that more studies say Drug X prevents stroke, therefore Drug X seems to be efficacious, these types of analyses factor in the quality and size of each study and other important factors. The Cochrane Collaboration (www.cochrane.org), mentioned in the final chapter, compiles these "super-studies" in one central website.

In addition, clinicians frequently rely on evidence-based practice guidelines to help guide prescribing and other areas of practice. These guidelines are typically prepared by experts in the field for professional associations and use information from meta analyses and systematic reviews.

All the above approaches factor in the design of the studies into their decision-making. For example, Study A, a large-scale randomized controlled trial, would be weighted differently than a single published report of a physician who describes what he observed in a single patient. This is not to discount case reports of physicians describing unique experiences of individual patients. However, factoring the quality of the study design does help clinicians and researchers compile the evidence to make better informed decisions under conditions where the evidence is conflicting. See "Following the Doughnut Trail" to read about a situation where the evidence was much clearer.

Following the Doughnut Trail

If only all evidence were so clear and led to such a quick resolution of a crime. When a doughnut deliveryman stopped at a convenience store to make a delivery and left the engine running, someone decided it was a great opportunity to make off with the truck. Unfortunately for the thief, the deliveryman had left the back doors of the truck open and the police literally followed a trail of doughnuts to easily find the stolen truck. As the police sergeant later said, "It has a happy ending. The evidence was brought back to the police station, and the cops are eating the doughnuts." Although he was joking about eating the evidence, the police were rewarded for solving the crime so quickly by receiving a special delivery of doughnuts to their station by the doughnut company.[136]

Our advice when you are faced with conflicting or unsettling information from the media about a drug you are taking is to speak to your physician and pharmacist. Don't make a rash decision based on one news report. Even in a worst-case scenario where new research has discovered a life-threatening side effect from an existing medication and the drug has been taken off the market by Health Canada, you should make an appointment with the physician who prescribed the medication to find out if you should be switched to a different medication or something else should be done. For some medications, it can be quite dangerous if they are abruptly stopped.

Specific Sources of Drug and Health-Care Information

Now that we have reviewed the process of drug discovery and how research on new drugs is generated and published, let's turn to specific sources of information. Many of these sources simply try to take the information from published clinical trials and phase iv research and interpret it. Others, such as a newspaper article reporting on a new promising drug, may only focus on a single trial without providing a larger context. Some drug and health-care information sources are compiled by medical experts, while others are not. While we couldn't possibly cover all sources in a book the size of *Take as Directed*, we will focus on some of the main sources for information you are likely to encounter.

The blue bible

If you have ever been to a doctor's office or to a pharmacy, and let's face it, who hasn't, there is a good chance you have seen a thick blue book either sitting on a desk or counter or being flipped through by the physician or pharmacist. This book, sometimes called "the blue bible," is officially known as the cps — the *Compendium of Pharmaceuticals and Specialties*. It is published annually by the Canadian Pharmacists Association, and a copy is provided for free to each physician in Canada and to pharmacists who are association members. It is now available in electronic format as well (the *e-CPS*). It can be purchased by anyone in either format at www.pharmacists.ca. Billed as "the Canadian drug reference for health professionals," it does seem to live up to its title, given how frequently it is used by these individuals.

So, what information is contained in this book and where does it come from? The bulk of the approximately 2,700 pages of the CPS consist of drug product monographs. These monographs, approved by Health Canada, are very detailed descriptions of drugs, containing such information as the pharmacology of the drug (how it works in the human body), indications (Health Canada–approved uses), contraindications (conditions where it should not be prescribed), warnings and precautions, adverse effects (side effects), and recommended dosing of the drug. A word of caution is that most side effects, no matter how infrequent, reported in clinical trials are included in the drug product monographs. Other sections of the CPS are primarily prepared by the editorial staff of the Canadian Pharmacists Association and include such things as photographs of commonly prescribed medications, a comprehensive directory of the nation's poison control centres, health organizations and pharmaceutical companies, and additional clinical information, including drug use in pregnancy and lactation, and drug interactions. There is definitely information in the CPS that will be of interest to the general public, although keep in mind that the book has been prepared with health professionals as the primary audience.

If you do not wish to purchase the entire book but would like to see the drug product monographs for the drugs you are taking, there are a few options available to you. First, you can freely access the official drug product monographs via the product's "entry" in Health Canada's drug product database (www.hc-sc.gc.ca/dhp-mps/prod-pharma/databasdon/index-eng.php). Second, the closest branch of your local public library may have a copy of the CPS, although you will want to make sure it is a recent edition. Third, we recommend asking your pharmacist to borrow a copy of the CPS to read while you are waiting to have your prescription filled or to ask your pharmacist to photocopy the relevant pages for you. Be forewarned — the font for the drug product monographs in the CPS is extremely small so you may want to purchase a magnifier at the pharmacy at the same time!

Printed information from the pharmacy

Another common source for drug information is the printed information that your pharmacist likely provides when you pick up your filled prescription. This information may be in the form of a sheet of paper, leaflet, or pamphlet, stapled to the prescription bag, placed inside the bag, or simply handed to you by the pharmacist. Ideally, the pharmacist will spend time with you reviewing this information, perhaps highlighting or circling critical points and crossing out the written information that does not apply to your situation. If your pharmacist does not provide verbal counselling in addition to the written information, we suggest you ask her to do this the next time you have your prescription filled.

If you take the time to read this information when you return home, you may be surprised how detailed the information typically is and how many side effects are listed. Similar to the drug product monographs in the CPS, the written information from a pharmacy tends to list almost every known side effect and errs on the side of providing comprehensive, and sometimes too much, information. In fact, it may cause you to wonder why you have been prescribed the drug at all after reading through all this information!

It may surprise you to learn that regardless of the pharmacy you go to, the information for most written information comes from the same third-party sources such as First Databank or Wolters Kluwer Health Inc. A report delivered to the U.S. Department of Health and Human Services and the Food and Drug Administration in 2008 was quite critical of the information contained in the written handouts from pharmacies. In this study, the printed information given to secret shoppers from more than 350 randomly selected pharmacies in the United States for two commonly prescribed drugs, lisinopril (used to treat heart disease and high blood pressure and to prevent diabetic kidney damage) and metformin (used to treat diabetes), was reviewed by a panel of experts. The number of words in the printed information received by these patients ranged from a low of 33 words to a high of 2,482 words. While the panel determined that the written information provided by these pharmacies did a good job of listing precautions and adverse reactions and was accurate, it scored poorly in other areas. The one area that scored the lowest was legibility and comprehensibility. Only 29% of the printed information leaflets were font size 10 or larger, while only 10% of lisinopril and 6% of metformin leaflets were written at or below an eighth grade reading level.[137] While a similar Canadian study has not been completed at the time of writing *Take as Directed*, the information given by Canadian community pharmacies typically comes from the same sources as those reviewed in this American study.

Our suggestion is to take some time to carefully read over the leaflet once you return home from the pharmacy. Try not to panic when you read these handouts and definitely don't decide not to take your prescription because you are scared of the potential side effects. If you have questions about what you have read, phone the pharmacist to discuss your questions or you may have more urgent concerns that require a conversation with your physician. If your pharmacy has scheduled a callback as we discussed in Chapter 6, this is also an ideal time to review your leaflet in more depth with your pharmacist.

Drug and health-care information on the internet

A challenge for us in writing *Take as Directed* was how to come up with a meaningful list of reputable websites for you to turn to for more information, given the dynamic, evolving nature of content on the internet and wide variety of diseases and drugs in which our readers may be interested. So, rather than creating a lengthy table with dozens of websites, we are recommending four specific websites as reputable entry points or portals through which you can begin your searches for drug and health-care information on the internet.

The first portal is Drug Information Resources: A Guide for Pharmacists (dir.pharmacy.dal.ca), actively maintained by the Dalhousie University College of Pharmacy. Don't be fooled by the title; besides being useful for pharmacists and other health professionals, it is also helpful for the general public. It may seem like favouritism to recommend a website associated with the employer of one of us (NM), but we can recommend this site as we have personally used it and it has been recognized internationally in the past as a great website for drug information.

The links to drug information sources on this website are regularly reviewed and updated by a team of health professionals and librarians. Moreover, this website itself has been certified by the Health on the Net Foundation as an ethical and trustworthy source of health information. There are too many categories of information on the website to review here, but examples of links include websites where you can check for drug interactions among your own medication and links to websites and books about medication safety. Likely of interest to many of you, there is a category called "Consumer Health," which contains links to websites for more information on health conditions and treatment information, information for patients from journals, and other topics. The website also indicates which resources are free.

Second, as we mentioned previously, the Health Canada website (www.hc-sc.gc.ca) contains a wealth of information. In addition to the Drug Product Database, this website includes health-care advisories, warnings, and recalls; general information on healthy living; and an in-depth section on consumer product safety, including products such as household cleaners and children's products. While the Health Canada website contains extremely valuable information, in, some would say, typical government fashion, parts of the website are not very user-friendly or easy to navigate.

Our third recommendation is MedlinePlus (www.nlm.nih.gov/medlineplus), a service of the U.S. National Library of Medicine and the U.S. National Institutes of Health designed for consumers. It contains written information on medications and health conditions, a link to the website for clinical trials we reviewed earlier in this chapter, as well as videos and slideshows. Keep in mind that it is an American website when reviewing the drug information as not all drugs approved for use in the United States have been approved for use in Canada and vice versa. This website also contains a tutorial on how to evaluate health information that you may find on the internet.

Our final recommendation is the Health Council of Canada's website (www.healthcouncilcanada.ca). This organization is our nation's health-care watchdog and produces reports on a regular basis aimed at the general public on a wide variety of health-care topics. You won't find information on drugs or treatments for specific diseases or conditions on this website, but rather information on issues such as the quality and safety of our health-care system and how money is being spent by our governments on various health-care initiatives. Examples of reports in recent years include disease management in Canadians with chronic illness, wait times, and home care. All its reports can be downloaded for free.

Other websites receiving an honourable mention from us include the Jewish General Hospital in Montreal (www.jgh.ca/en/HerzlGeneralHealth) and the websites for the provincial and territorial departments of health. Finally, it is always a great idea to discuss any information you find on the internet, whether through our recommended websites or another source, with your physician and pharmacist.

Conclusion

The advent of the Information Age has been both a blessing and a curse for those interested in health-care information. On one hand, learning more about one's diseases and drugs is easier than ever before and does not require a trip to the back aisle of your local library and dusting off possibly out-of-date medical textbooks. On the other hand, it is difficult to know whether to trust the information you are reading and how to deal with seemingly conflicting information. We hope this chapter has helped to demystify drug and health-care information and gets your search for more information started in the right direction.

CHAPTER ELEVEN

PRESCRIBING A BRIGHTER FUTURE FOR HEALTH CARE

A Blueprint for Change

In this final chapter of *Take as Directed,* we present some suggestions for improving the safety and quality of health care in Canada. Many of these recommendations are specifically targeted toward the medication-use system. Some of the recommendations are directed to health-care decision-makers — politicians, government agencies, CEOs of hospitals and health authorities, and health professional thought leaders. While some of these recommendations may seem out of reach for you as a health-care consumer, it's important to remember that many of the decision-makers such as politicians work for and are elected by you or, as bureaucrats, are accountable to the general public. When they are looking for your support, it's worth asking your political candidates how they would work toward developing a catastrophic drug plan, for example.

Other recommendations are directed toward you, the reader, since we believe that real change and a culture of improved safety in our health-care system must include those who use it. In most cases, our recommendations build upon ideas we've previously introduced in *Take as Directed.*

We have tried to refrain from ending this book with a rant. Yes, it is easy to criticize the health-care system as there are many areas in which safety, quality, or access could be improved. At the same time, we are proud of our health-care system and we believe that it meets the needs of a majority of Canadians, particularly when they are very ill. Recent national surveys indicate that most Canadians are either satisfied or very satisfied with our health-care system. So please consider our recommendations as vital tweaks rather than a complete rebuild of health care in Canada.

Finally, we will end the chapter with a discussion of the nature of change in health care and leave you with some examples of how change is possible.

A Catastrophic Drug Plan — And Then Some

William, a resident of Western Canada, was diagnosed with lymphoma the week before his sixty-seventh birthday. He was relieved to know that he would not need to be treated in hospital for his cancer and that his provincial health plan would pick up the $62,000-a-year cost of the medication his oncologist recommended. He and his wife had one grown daughter who lived on the East Coast, and they had often talked about retiring there in order to be closer to her and her family. After his diagnosis, they felt the desire to move more acutely as William's oncologist had indicated the treatment he was receiving would prolong his life but would not cure the cancer. However, after making inquiries, William learned that the cost of his cancer medication would not be covered in the new province. Ultimately, he and his wife made the difficult decision to stay in their home province.

One of the existing barriers to receiving optimum health care is the inability to pay for necessary treatment, particularly drug treatment. As we have seen, the Canada Health Act covers only services provided in hospitals or by physicians. Drugs administered in a hospital are covered but those taken at home by the patient are not. The Canadian Cancer Society's report on catastrophic drug coverage released in

September 2009 says that eleven of the twenty new cancer-treating medications released since 2000 are taken in the home by the patient, meaning that the patient must bear the costs of the drugs, which average $65,000 a year. The report also states that 6% of all Canadians pay in excess of $1,000 a year in drug costs and one in twelve families spends in excess of 3% of its annual net income on medications.[138] Governments and third-party payers, for their part, are left grappling with which costly drugs to cover, knowing that many of them prolong a cancer patient's life by just a few weeks.

In the early 2000s, the Canadian government commissioned former Saskatchewan premier Roy Romanow to examine the state of the Canadian health-care system and to make recommendations regarding the future of health-care delivery in the nation. Romanow released his report "Building on Values: The Future of Health Care in Canada" in November 2002. Among his key recommendations was that a catastrophic drug transfer fund be established to allow the provinces and territories to enhance coverage for residents facing catastrophic drug costs. Two years later, the National Pharmaceuticals Strategy was announced to look at the issue of access to medications, in addition to affordability, quality, and safety, but this process has stalled. As we go to print, most provinces and territories have moved ahead on their own and provided some degree of coverage for individuals facing catastrophic drug costs, but the coverage is far from universal and varies widely from one area of the country to another. Some costs are borne by private insurers, who commonly put a ceiling on the costs they are willing to cover. Many require the patient to pay 20% of the drug costs, which can still amount to tens of thousands of dollars a year.

For more on the National Pharmaceuticals Strategy, we recommend the companion reports by the Health Council of Canada that were released in 2009 and are available for free on its website (www.healthcouncilcanada.ca). The reports are written in a non-technical, engaging writing style and show the progress, or lack thereof, made by our federal, provincial, and territorial governments on the nine components of the National Pharmaceuticals Strategy. We also support the Health Council of Canada's recommendation for moving forward on this important issue as outlined in its reports.[139]

Public catastrophic drug coverage is inconsistent across the nation and there are many gaps. For example, workers in New Brunswick and Prince Edward Island who do not have third-party insurance through their jobs are not eligible for publicly funded coverage. In some provinces, higher income residents are not eligible for catastrophic drug coverage at all or must pay prohibitively high deductibles. The problem of lack of access to coverage is particularly acute in Atlantic Canada, with significant gaps in coverage for many seniors as well as those who do not belong to low-income groups. This is clearly an area in dire need of attention.

However, it is not only the drugs costing tens of thousands of dollars a year that can lead to financial hardship. For many Canadians, even more modestly priced drugs may be difficult to afford. Many individuals faced with drug costs beyond their means will simply not take the drug, or not take it as it was prescribed, thereby increasing the risks of a less-than-optimum outcome. Just as coverage for catastrophic drugs is a patchwork across the country, so, too, is coverage for more mainstream drugs. Although spending on drugs represents the fastest-growing cost within the health-care system, only Quebec requires its residents to have either public or private (e.g., employee) insurance to cover the cost of prescribed medications. In our vision for the future, there will be a cohesive pan-Canadian approach to both catastrophic and mainstream drug costs and all Canadians will have the right not to have to face financial hardship because of the cost of necessary medication.

A Family Physician for Every Canadian

As we saw in Chapter 2, individuals who didn't have a regular doctor were more likely to report that they had experienced an adverse event during an encounter with the health-care system. In our vision for the future, every Canadian will have a family physician to call his or her own. In order to realize this vision, we believe a three-pronged approach is needed.

- **First, medical school enrolments need to continue to increase.** As planning for the number of needed medical school seats takes place, policy-makers must consider the feminization of the medical workforce and trend among younger physicians toward more sane work hours than their predecessors.
- **Second, we need to roll out the welcome mat to the thousands** of Canadians who are currently receiving, or have received, medical training in other parts of the world. Because of the shortage of medical school seats, many talented and bright Canadian students have difficulty securing a spot in one of our medical schools and instead obtain their degrees in another country. After completing their training, many never return to Canada, laying down roots instead in the country where they trained. A plan to improve access to physicians in this country, therefore, must include a plan to repatriate these physicians, many of whom are just beginning their careers.
- **Third, we need to look at ways to streamline assessment** of the skills of international medical graduates who are not Canadian by birth but are now living in this country. We believe that Canada should aim to become self-sufficient in producing enough physicians to meet our needs as a nation, and not rely on poaching physicians from other parts of the world that can ill afford to lose them. A plan to expedite the assessment of the skills of physician immigrants to Canada and assist them into the transition into medical practice in our country is much needed. While advances are being made in a number of areas of the country, there is still work to be done in order to tap this huge reservoir of available medical personnel.

Enough Face Time with the Doctor

Individuals who report that they don't have enough "face time" with their doctor are more likely to report they experienced an adverse health outcome or error. The key to ensuring that physicians have adequate time to address patient needs involves looking at new models of care — and rethinking the way that Canadian doctors have traditionally been paid.

In many places, health-care teams share in the care of the patient, with each member of the team responsible for that aspect of the patient's care to which he or she is best able. For example, a registered nurse or a nurse practitioner might perform health-maintenance manoeuvres such as Pap tests, blood pressure monitoring, well-baby examinations, and immunizations. A registered dietician might provide counselling regarding weight reduction, cholesterol lowering, or diabetes management or to a patient who has dietary restrictions as a result of chronic kidney disease. A pharmacist might provide counselling on proper medication use. In these teams, the physician focuses on managing individuals with complex medical issues. These collaborative care teams have earned high marks from both members of the teams who staff them, as well as from patients themselves, and evidence is emerging that patient outcomes are improved when patients receive such team-based care. However, in order for this model to succeed, there must be a movement away from the traditional fee-for-service remuneration models for physician payment, as well as for other members of the team. Currently, focusing on management of complex illness is not sustainable as a business model in family practice, where physicians have needed to rely on seeing a certain number of individuals with minor illnesses in order to cover the increasing overhead costs associated with running a practice. Having minor illnesses and health-prevention manoeuvres such as immunizations and Pap tests performed by other members of the team sounds like a good idea, but it will only work if physician remuneration models reflect the additional time needed to care for a patient with complex health issues. This is beginning to happen in a number of jurisdictions, and additionally physicians in some provinces now receive incentives for meeting targets such as offering flu shots, discussing smoking cessation, and ensuring that their diabetic patients receive annual foot and eye examinations. Incentives such as these will help to improve health outcomes for residents of these provinces with chronic disease who do need more "face time" with their doctor and other members of the health-care team. They should also help to improve the business model for the family physician providing cradle-to-grave care, which should lead to improved access to family physicians for Canadians.

Electronic Health Records

As we have said throughout this book, one of the commonest places in which adverse health-care outcomes arise is during transitions from one health-care setting to another. At these transitions, critical information about the patient may not be available to a new provider or team of providers. Thinking back to Paul, the recently retired man in our introductory chapter who developed near-fatal rhabdomyolysis because of an interaction between an antibiotic and a cholesterol-lowering medication, we can identify some of these information gaps. Paul was cared for by both a physician and a pharmacist who were unfamiliar to him and neither was aware of the long-term medications he was taking.

At this time, information about our personal health commonly exists in silos, only available to the person or persons caring for us at that particular location. The record our family physician keeps is available at his or her clinic but is not usually available to the doctor at the local emergency department or the pharmacist who fills our prescription. When our family doctor refers us to a specialist, he or she sends along the parts of our health record that are relevant, but this information may be illegible or even outdated by the time we see the specialist. Of course, we do not want every single health-care provider we see to have access to all our medical information. For example, it is unnecessary for our eye doctor to have the details of our last gynecologic examination or of the time we saw a mental health professional regarding marital difficulties. However, lack of up-to-date information available to those caring for us can have serious consequences. It is unfathomable that for all our advances in biotechnology, such as our ability over the last generation to cure many cancers that were once lethal and identify the precise chromosomal aberration that causes many diseases, we still have a health-care system that is held together by an antiquated system of paperwork.

Electronic health records (EHRs) have many safety advantages over traditional paper charts, including identification of interactions between medications, "at a glance" medication lists, and features that alert a physician if he or she attempts to prescribe a medication to which the patient is allergic. However, information contained within them is only available at that point of care; interconnectedness of health information between locales where care is provided remains an issue. For example, if your family doctor uses an electronic record, chances are that the physician who sees you at the walk-in clinic or the emergency department cannot access those records. And if your hospital maintains electronic records, chances are they can't be viewed by your family doctor. Currently, records that are generated as a result of a hospital visit are likely only to be able to be seen in that province — meaning that the doctor seeing you on an emergency basis in Alberta may be unable to quickly access the results of the CT scan you had to monitor your aneurysm in New Brunswick.

Clearly, Canadians deserve a health record that will allow caregivers in a variety of locations to access those parts of your health record that they need in order to care for you. Canada Health Infoway is a not-for-profit organization that works with governments, health-care providers, and other stakeholders to promote and accelerate the use of electronic health records across the country.

Thus far, Infoway's focus has been on institutional settings, with less investment in physician offices where much of the health care in Canada is provided. Although important work has begun, continued investment is needed in order to realize the Infoway vision of an interconnected Canadian EHR network from sea to sea to sea.

Additionally, as discussed in Chapter 9, Canadians themselves should be able to maintain and access electronic health records of their own. Websites such as Google Health, which allow individuals to do just that, are clearly a sign of things to come.

Engage Patients in Safety and Quality Activities

Our next recommendation is to engage patients in activities that are known to improve the safety and/or quality of health care in Canada. At first glance, this may seem like a fairly vague suggestion that would be hard to implement. Delving deeper, what might this look like at a practical level?

A study in the Midwestern United States provides a glimpse of how this might work. In this study, telephone interviews were conducted with more than 2,000 patients who were recently discharged from one of eleven participating hospitals. The patients were asked a series of questions about their comfort level in performing error prevention behaviours and whether they actually performed those behaviours during their hospitalization.

The following table contains the seven error prevention behaviours. What is striking is that for several of the behaviours, such as asking the nurse the purpose of the medication, asking questions about medical care, and telling the medical staff an error occurred, patients said they were *both* very comfortable performing those behaviours *and* did take action. For several other behaviours, such as asking the nurse to confirm the patient's identity, having a family member or friend watch for errors, and helping health professionals mark the surgical location, the patients said they were very comfortable performing that behaviour but for some reason they failed to take action and did not actually perform the behaviour when given the opportunity. Finally, for one other behaviour, asking medical personnel whether they washed their hands, less than half of patients said they were very comfortable performing that behaviour while only about one in twenty patients actually took action and performed the behaviour when given the opportunity.

The Comfort Level of Patients in Performing Error Prevention Behaviours[140]

Error Prevention Behaviour	% Very Comfortable	% Patients Who Took Action
Ask nurse purpose of medication	91.3	75.2
Ask questions about medical care	88.8	85.1
Ask nurse to confirm patient's identity	84.2	37.8
Tell medical staff that error occurred	78.4	79.7
Have family member or friend watch for errors	76.0	38.6
Help health professionals mark surgical location	71.5	17.3
Ask medical personnel whether they washed their hands	45.5	4.6

Note: Only patients who were asked about the behaviour and had the opportunity to perform the behaviour while hospitalized were included.

What this study suggests is that patients are comfortable performing many error prevention behaviours that are known to improve safety and quality. However, there are other error prevention behaviours that patients will need encouragement to perform. Some of the solutions may be quite simple, such as having pharmacists wear buttons that read, "Ask me about your medications" or presenting patients and their families with a list of suggested error prevention strategies upon admission to a hospital or long-term care facility. There are limits to patient engagement, of course — not all patients will have the capacity to participate in these behaviours (such as patients in a coma), and we certainly don't want to cause patients unnecessary alarm about the possibility of experiencing a preventable adverse event. Nonetheless, it is clear there is a potentially much larger role for patients to play and thus we have included this in our list of recommendations.

Develop a National Information System for Health-Care Safety and Quality

Imagine this: A surgical team logs onto a computer and quickly reviews all the adverse events that have occurred across the country in the past month in other hospitals for the same type of surgical procedure and discusses how, as a team, to avoid similar adverse events. A family physician is considering prescribing a new drug for the first time and logs on to a computer to review commonly reported errors with that medication, all adverse drug reactions that have been reported by patients and health professionals across Canada, and how the cost of this new medication compares to existing similar drugs. A patient moves to a new community and logs on to a computer to see which pharmacies in town offer blood pressure clinics and medication reviews.

Ideally, the above scenarios should exist in Canada today. Parts of the above scenarios exist in other countries. As we have already reviewed in this chapter, the Canada Health Infoway is making progress toward implementing electronic health records, but there is much more that could be done to improve the safety and quality of our health-care system. For example, while each hospital in Canada has its own reporting system for adverse events as we reviewed in Chapter 9, there is currently no national system that collects and analyzes all adverse events from hospitals, pharmacies, physician offices, clinics, long-term care facilities, emergency response teams, and other health-care settings. Health Canada has set up a system called MedEffect Canada where Canadians can report side effects to medication, but at the time of writing this book, there is no place where Canadians can report errors and other preventable adverse events easily. Many systems, some of which overlap, are in various stages of development, such as the National System for Incident Reporting, the Canadian Medication Incident Reporting and Prevention System program, the Canadian Adverse Event Reporting and Learning System, and the Drug Safety and Effectiveness Network. Many of these systems are years away from fully being implemented, and even when fully developed there will still be gaps and a lack of easily accessible shared information for both health professionals and patients alike.

We recommend a single information warehouse that includes adverse events from all health-care settings reported by patients, health professionals, and risk managers, which can be accessed online by anyone in Canada. Needless to say, such an initiative would require significant human and financial resources but would serve to greatly improve the safety and quality of our health-care system.

A Known Goal with Each Prescription

Let's move from a complex strategy to a simple and inexpensive recommendation. What is this recommendation? We suggest that each prescription has clear, measurable goals and that these are known by the prescriber, the pharmacist, and the patient (and caregiver) along with any other relevant health professionals. In short, all the above individuals should be able to answer the question "What is the goal we are trying to achieve with this Rx?" To put it another way, if one or more of the above individuals do not know the purpose of the medication, why was it prescribed in the first place?

We also want to clarify what we mean by the goal or purpose of the medication. By this, we are not referring to a vague response such as "for high blood pressure" or "for asthma." Medications often have different uses, and it may surprise you that sometimes the community pharmacist does not even known the basic use of the medication for a specific patient when filling a prescription. A more appropriate goal than "for asthma" might be the goal for Elliott, a teenaged boy with asthma, to be able to play soccer with his team without wheezing and getting winded. Another appropriate goal would be to reduce the number of trips Elliott makes to the emergency department with an exacerbation of asthma from the number of trips last year. These are measurable goals that can be tracked over time. Setting specific targets such as these will help the prescriber, the patient, and caregivers know whether the medication is achieving its intended purpose. If Elliott made three trips to the emergency department last year due to asthma and has already made five trips through the first six months of this year, it is a good indication that the medication is not achieving its intended purpose and that some type of change needs to be made, such as increasing the dosage, prescribing a different medication, and so on. Moreover, when the pharmacist is privy to the specific goals, he or she can help the patient monitor therapy in between physician office visits and also more effectively check for appropriate dosage and other drug-related problems when filling a prescription. As we move to electronic health records in Canada that include personal health records, ideally the goal of each prescribed medication will be included and easily accessible by the prescriber, pharmacist, and patient. Until we reach that point, our recommendation for you, the reader, is to make sure you have written down the specific goal for each of your medications. If you are unsure of the goal, please speak to the physician who prescribed that medication.

Implement Best Demonstrated Practices

As you would likely agree, there are many areas in health care where new research is urgently needed. These areas include cures for existing diseases, newly improved surgical and diagnostic techniques, or simply finding less expensive ways of doing things. At the same time, many would argue that another strategy that would vastly improve the safety and quality of health care would be for the findings of existing studies and reports to be fully implemented. For example, as we reviewed earlier in this chapter, we are still waiting for the recommendations in the "Building on Values: The Future of Health Care in Canada" report and the National Pharmaceuticals Strategy to be implemented.

In his book *Patients First*, Canadian physician Dr. Terrence Montague calls these gaps between study results and resulting improvements to health care "care gaps," and he gives many examples of where best demonstrated practices in health care have not been fully implemented. For example, he touches on the underuse of drugs such as ASA (Aspirin) and beta-blockers in patients who have experienced a heart attack.[141] These drugs help to prevent a second heart attack and yet are under-prescribed in patients who have experienced a heart attack in Canada. Care gaps may not be as exciting or grab the headlines like the results of a promising new drug or procedure, but the health-care literature suggests that these gaps are the norm rather than the exception and that we would be wise to spend more resources on trying to implement the findings of existing research rather than launching yet another study.

Often considerable effort is placed in clinical trials to develop new drugs or new guidelines to help physicians and other health professionals practise more effectively, only to see these drugs used inappropriately or the guidelines not followed by clinicians in the real world.

The good news is that there are some organizations that collect the best evidence to improve quality and safety and are actively working to have it implemented in health care. Some of these organizations and initiatives include the Cochrane Collaboration (www.cochrane.org) and the Canadian Agency for Drugs and Technologies in Health (www.cadth.ca). Many Canadian health-care research funding agencies, including the Canadian Institutes of Health Research, are also now funding what is known as *knowledge translation* — efforts to speed the uptake of new research into actual health-care practice. The theory is that if in the past it often took a decade or longer to have the results from a new study fully implemented and we can shorten this to five years or fewer, we can significantly improve health care.

The literature also suggests that once a critical mass of health professionals change practice and adopt a new procedure or use a new guideline, a tipping point is reached and the majority of practice changes. This may be due in part to peer pressure, patient or payer expectations, or other reasons. We see this in all industries, of course, whether it is the adoption of a new corn hybrid among farmers or DVD players.

Another analogy is that "a rising tide lifts all boats." That is, once there is a tide (i.e., adoption of a new guideline, etc.), the impact will be felt by all. Those residents of New Brunswick and Nova Scotia who live along the Bay of Fundy are well aware of the impact of the tide and how all boats — whether a small dory or large container ship — will be equally impacted by the rising or lowering tide. In our case, the rising tide may be new disclosure guidelines for health professionals for reporting errors or a drug recall by Health Canada. Such a change will impact all clinicians.

Another piece of good news is that for the medication-use system, in particular, the best demonstrated practices are known. As we reviewed in Chapter 2, there are eight essential elements of a safe and effective medication-use system, and most adverse drug events occur because one or more of the elements were not in place for a given patient. This is, in essence, the care gap for the medication-use system and effort can then be placed on closing this gap. If the eight essential elements of a safe and effective medication-use system were fully implemented for each Canadian, there would be a considerable impact on adverse drug events.

Conclusion: Implement Change in Health Care

While we have presented eight recommendations for improving Canada's health-care system in this chapter, a skeptic could argue that it is easy to propose solutions; it is the implementation part that is tricky. Indeed, this is probably all the more true in health care where one is dealing with longstanding health professional bodies and organizations, all with a vested interest in protecting the status quo and viewing change with suspicion. Implementing change can be very, very hard in health care, regardless of the country of origin, as we have recently witnessed with the health reform debate south of the border.

Still, we hope that the magnitude of the problems we have addressed in this book will bring some urgency to the situation. On one hand, problems related to lack of knowledge, poor quality, safety, lack of affordability and access have been with us for a long, long time. On the other hand, new evidence has emerged in recent years that we have reviewed in *Take as Directed* that describes the preventable harm to patients and needless costs to the health-care system due to adverse events and other problems.

A couple of real-world examples show the challenge of fostering change in health care, even when the evidence is on your side.

Fighting the medical establishment one baby at a time
The first example involves a physician in Vienna who lived from 1818 to 1865, Ignaz Semmelweis.[142] Dr. Semmelweis is not exactly a household name today, but what he did certainly revolutionized health care in one area. In his day, childbirth fever was a major cause of death in new mothers. Moreover, "unbelievable as it seems, professors and their students in medical universities went from the dissecting room, where they demonstrated and practised delivering babies from cadavers, to the Lying In rooms where they examined women about to give birth — all without washing or disinfecting their hands. A gratuitous rubbing of their bloody hands on their lab coats was considered ample readiness, and in fact the presence of bloody matter on their coats was deemed almost a badge of honour."[143] Dr. Semmelweis began to use handwashing and the use of an antiseptic solution (chlorinated lime) with his patients and wisely took detailed measurements of their impact on mortality and published his findings.

Unfortunately, despite the evidence Dr. Semmelweis accumulated, the medical community was not convinced. His boss, Dr. Klein, told him: "Keep yourself to what is old, for that is good. If our ancestors have proven it to be good, why should we not do as they did? Mistrust new ideas. I have no need of learned men. I need faithful subjects. He who would serve me must do what I command. He who cannot do this or who comes full of new ideas may go his way. If he does not, I shall send him. Do you understand, Dr. Semmelweis?"[144] This sounds like the kind of boss we'd all like to have, right? Dr. Semmelweis died at the age of forty-seven in an asylum, never seeing the widespread implementation of his research.

A pain in the gut

This story about Dr. Semmelweis could be easily dismissed as an artifact of a health-care community long passed. However, a more recent example shows that changing health care remains equally as difficult in modern times.

In 1979, Robin Warren, a pathologist at a hospital in Australia, discovered a bacterium in biopsies from patients who had stomach inflammation. His initial reports were rejected by the medical community, as it was thought that no bacteria could live in the stomach due to the acidic nature of this environment. Still, he pressed on with additional research in partnership with a gastroenterologist, Dr. Barry Marshall.[145]

Over the next few years they discovered that this bacterium, which they named *Helicobacter pylori*, was present in a large majority of patients with stomach inflammation or ulcers. They published more results in the medical journal *The Lancet* but were still greeted by skepticism from the medical community. Finally, in order to show what happened when infected by this bacterium, Dr. Marshall swallowed a culture of the bacterium, developed severe acute stomach inflammation, and documented this process. In the following years, Drs. Marshall and Warren would show how the use of antibiotics successfully treated ulcers. Over time, their results became accepted by the medical community, and now fortunately peptic ulcers have moved from being a chronic and painful condition to something that can be cured by a short course of antibiotics and other drugs. In 2005, Drs. Marshall and Warren received the Nobel Prize in Physiology or Medicine.[146]

How, Then, Do We Change Health Care?

Given the challenges in changing health-care practice, how can we move forward with the ideas expressed in this book? One way to think about changing health-care practice can be seen in the following table. In this 2 x 2 table, one can view the item in question — whether it be one of our eight recommendations, the widespread adoption of prescribing of a new drug or procedure, or another health-care issue, as already being in health-care practice or not. Next, one can think about new research that either has positive results (saves lives, reduces health-care costs, etc.) or negative results (kills patients, results in harm, etc.). Let's review each of the quadrants in turn.

Implementing Change in Health-Care Practice

	New Research — Positive Results	New Research — Negative Results
Already in health-care practice	Quadrant I: Change not needed (or small change needed)	Quadrant II: Change is hard or easy.
Not already in health-care practice	Quadrant III: Change is hard!	Quadrant IV: Change not needed (but hard to get study published)

In Quadrant I, where a new study comes out with positive results about something we're already doing in health care, typically little change if any is needed. For example, this may be the latest in a long series of studies that has found that Drug X will help patients with Condition Y. It is helpful to have new studies that confirm what we already know, although this new study will likely have little impact on health-care practice.

In Quadrant II, where a new study comes out with negative results about something we're already doing in health care, the change can be easy or hard. It may surprise you that sometimes the change is hard, but if it is a practice that is well engrained in health care and the study has some flaws, it may not be enough to change practice. Sometimes the change will occur gradually over time as well.

In Quadrant III, where a new study comes out with positive results about something we're not doing already in health care, the change is typically hard. Both of our examples — Dr. Semmelweis, handwashing and use of antiseptic solutions, and Drs. Marshall and Warren and the use of antibiotics to treat ulcers — fit into this category. In addition, most of our eight recommendations fall into this category.

Finally, in Quadrant IV, where a new study comes out with negative results about something we're not doing already in health care, typically change is not needed. Moreover, health-care journal editors are usually not very excited to publish studies in this quadrant.

We should also acknowledge that sometimes there is a perfect alignment of events and timing is the overriding factor. Read "Is There a Doctor or Fifteen on Board?" for such an event.

Is There a Doctor or Fifteen on Board?

Is timing everything? For Dorothy Fletcher it certainly was. On a mid-Atlantic flight from the United Kingdom to Orlando, Florida, the cabin crew asked if there was a doctor on board after one of the passengers, a sixty-seven-year-old woman, Dorothy Fletcher, suffered a heart attack. Luckily, fifteen cardiologists, all on their way to a medical conference in Florida, pressed their call-bells and came to Dorothy's aid. They helped her to survive by giving her oxygen, monitored her blood pressure and pulse, and used an onboard medical kit to set up an intravenous infusion to thin her blood. As Mrs. Fletcher later remarked, "I couldn't believe what happened. All these people came rushing down the aircraft towards me. The doctors were wonderful. They saved my life. If there was ever a flight on which to have a heart attack, this was the one."[147]

Final Thoughts

We hope that you do not feel overwhelmed by the challenges in fostering change in health care. Change can happen. One reason we wanted to write this book is that we feel change can occur with you, one patient at a time. It is our belief that engaged and empowered individuals can improve the safety and quality of their own health-care experience and that of others as well.

NOTES

—

Chapter 1

1 Baker G.R., Norton P.G., Flintoft V. et al. 2004. "The Canadian Adverse Events Study: The Incidence of Adverse Events Among Hospital Patients in Canada." *Canadian Medical Association Journal* 170:1678–86.

2 Reason J. 2000. "Human Error: Models and Management." *British Medical Journal* 320:768–70. doi: 10.1136/bmj.320.7237.768.

3 Cadieux G., Tamblyn R., Dauphinee D., Libman M. 2007. "Predictors of Inappropriate Antibiotic Prescribing Among Primary Care Physicians." *Canadian Medical Association Journal* 177:877–883.

Chapter 2

4 Davies J.M., Hebert P., Hoffman C. 2003. *Canadian Patient Safety Dictionary.* Ottawa, ON: Royal College of Physicians and Surgeons of Canada. Available from: http://rcpsc.medical.org/publications/PatientSafetyDictionary_e.pdf.

5 MacKinnon N.J., U D., Koczmara C. 2008. "Medication Incidents Involving Heparin in Canada: 'Flushing' Out the Problem." *Canadian Journal of Hospital Pharmacy* 61(5):348–50.

6 Baker G.R., Jeffs L., Law M., Norton P.G. 2007. "Improving the Safety and Quality of Health Care in Canada." In MacKinnon N.J., ed., *Safe and Effective: The Eight Essential Elements of an Optimal Medication-Use System.* Ottawa, ON: Canadian Pharmacists Association.

7 Baker G.R., Norton P.G., Flintoft V. et al. 2004. "The Canadian Adverse Events Study: The Incidence of Adverse Events Among Hospital Patients in Canada." *Canadian Medical Association Journal* 170:1678–86.

8 Baker G.R., Jeffs L., Law M., Norton P.G. 2007. "Improving the Safety and Quality of Health Care in Canada." In MacKinnon N.J., ed., *Safe and Effective: The Eight Essential Elements of an Optimal Medication-Use System.* Ottawa, ON: Canadian Pharmacists Association.

9 Forster A.J., Clark H.D., Menard A. et al. 2004. "Adverse Events Among Medical Patients After Discharge from Hospital." *Canadian Medical Association Journal* 170:345–49.

10 Nickerson A., MacKinnon N.J., Roberts N., Saulnier L. 2005. "Drug-Therapy Problems, Inconsistencies and Omissions Identified During a Medication Reconciliation and Seamless Care Service." *Healthcare Quarterly* 8:65–72.

11 Schoen C., Osborn R., Doty M.M. et al. 2007. "Toward Higher-Performance Health Systems: Adult's Health Care Experiences in Seven Countries." *Health Affairs* 26(6):w717–w734.

12 MacKinnon N.J. 2008. "Could 7 Million Australians and Canadians Be Wrong? A Status Report on Medication-Use Safety in Australia and Canada" (editorial). *Journal of Pharmacy Practice and Research* 38(1):5–6.

13 Schoen C. et al. 2007.

14 Canadian Institute for Health Information. 2006. *Health Care in Canada Survey,* 2006. Ottawa, ON: CIHI.

15 O'Hagan J., MacKinnon N.J., Persaud D., Etchegary H. 2009. "Self-Reported Medical Errors in Seven Countries: Implications for Canada." *Healthcare Quarterly* 12 (Patient Safety Papers):55–61.

16 Ibid.

17 Scobie A.C., MacKinnon N.J., Higgins S.D., Etchegary H., Church R. 2009. "The Medical Home in Canada: Patient Perceptions of Quality and Safety." *Healthcare Management FORUM* 22(1):47–51.

18 MacKinnon N.J., Ip I. 2009. "The National Pharmaceuticals Strategy: Rest in Peace, Revive or Renew?" *Canadian Medical Association Journal* 180(8):801–3.

19 Canadian Institute for Health Information. 2010. "Drug Expenditure In Canada, 1985 to 2009." Ottawa, ON: CIHI.

20 Morgan S., Raymond C., Mooney D., Martin D. 2008. *The Canadian Rx Atlas*, 2nd ed. Vancouver, B.C.: University of British Columbia.

21 Ibid.

22 Ibid.

23 Ibid.

24 Morrison A., MacKinnon N.J., Hartnell N.R., McCaffrey K.J. 2008. "Impact of Drug Plan Management Policies in Canada: A Systematic Review." *Canadian Pharmacists Journal* 141(6):332–338.

25 Morgan S. et al. 2008.

26 "Politicians, Bureaucrats Enjoy Full Coverage of Drugs Not Covered in Public Plans." Available at http://www.50plus.com/Health/BrowseAllArticles/index.cfm?documentID=16760 www.carp.ca/display.cfm?CabinetID=263&LibraryID=70&cityID=7&documentI D=2244; Galloway G. January 23, 2007. "MPs' Drug Plan Beats Coverage for Elderly, Poor." *Globe and Mail.*

27 MacKinnon N.J., ed. 2007. *Safe and Effective: The Eight Essential Elements of an Optimal Medication-Use System*. Ottawa, ON: Canadian Pharmacists Association.

28 MacKinnon N.J. 2002. "Early Warning System: How Vigilant Pharmacists Can Prevent Drug-Related Morbidity in Seniors." *Pharmacy Practice* 18(8):40–4.

29 Johnson J.A., Bootman J.L. 1995. "Drug-Related Morbidity and Mortality. A Cost-of-Illness Model." *Archives of Internal Medicine* 155:1949–56.

30 Ernst F.R., Grizzle A.J. 2001. "Drug-Related Morbidity and Mortality: Updating the Cost-of-Illness Model." *Journal of the American Pharmacists Association* 41:192–99.

31 Bootman J.L., Harrison D.L., Cox E. 1997. "The Health Care Cost of Drug-Related Morbidity and Mortality in Nursing Facilities. *Archives of Internal Medicine* 157:2089–96.

32 Kidney T, MacKinnon N.J. 2001. "Preventable Drug-Related Morbidity and Mortality in Older Adults: A Canadian Cost-of-Illness Model." *Geriatrics Today* 4:120.

33 MacKinnon N.J., U D., Koczmara C. 2008. "Medication Incidents Involving Heparin in Canada: 'Flushing' Out the Problem." *Canadian Journal of Hospital Pharmacy* 61(5):348–50.

Chapter 3

34 Barer, M.L., Stoddart, G.L. 1991: "Toward Integrated Medical Resource Policies for Canada." Vancouver, BC: Centre for Health Services and Policy Research.

Chapter 4

35 Health Canada. 2007. "Recommendations for the Appropriate Use of Cough and Cold Products in Children." Available at www.hc-sc.gc.ca/ahc-asc/media/advisories-avis/_2007/2007_147_e.html.[0]

Health Canada. 2008. "Health Canada Released Decision on the Labelling of Cough and Cold Products for Children." Available at http://www.hc-sc.gc.ca/ahc-asc/media/advisories-avis/_2008/2008_184-eng.php.[0]

Canadian Paediatric Society. 2009. "Using Over-the-Counter Drugs to Treat Cold Symptoms." Available at www.caringforkids.cps.ca/whensick/OTC_Drugs.htm.

36 Canadian Paediatric Society. 2009. "Using Over-the-Counter Drugs to Treat Cold Symptoms." Available at www.caringforkids.cps.ca/whensick/OTC_Drugs.htm.

37 Peterson I., Johnson A.M., Islam A., Duckworth G., Livermore D.M., Hayward A.C. 2007. "Protective Effect of Antibiotics Against Serious Complications of Common Respiratory Tract Infections: Retrospective Cohort Study with the UK General Practice Research Database." *British Medical Journal* 335(76–27):982–987.

Chapter 5

38 Beckman H.B., Frankel R.M. 1984. "The Effect of Physician Behavior on the Collection of Data." *Annals of Internal Medicine* 101:692–6.

39 Langewitz W., Denz M., Keller A., Kiss A., Ruttimann S., Wossmer B. 2002. "Spontaneous Talking Time at Start of Consultation in Outpatient Clinic: Cohort Study." *British Medical Journal* 325:682–3. [o]

40 Shang A., Huwiler-Muntener K., Nartey L. et al. 2005. "Are the Clinical Effects of Homoeopathy Placebo Effects? Comparative Study of Placebo-Controlled Trials of Homoeopathy and Allopathy." *The Lancet* 366:726–32.

Chapter 6

41 IMS Health Canada. 2009. Available at www.imshealthcanada.com.

42 The Pharmacy Group. 2008. *Community Pharmacy in Canada: Executive Summary*. Toronto, ON: Rogers Business and Professional Publishing.

43 IMS Health Canada. 2009.

44 The Pharmacy Group. 2008.

45 Chang F. 2007. "Entering the Medication-Use System and Dealing with Drug-Related Problems." In MacKinnon N.J., ed., *Safe and Effective: The Eight Essential Elements of an Optimal Medication-Use System*. Ottawa, ON: Canadian Pharmacists Association.

46 Hepler C.D., Strand L. 1990. "Opportunities and Responsibilities in Pharmaceutical Care." *American Journal of Health-System Pharmacy* 47(3): 533–543.

47 Based on a modified version of a table in the following reference: Makowsky M.J., Tsuyuki R.T. 2007. "Pharmaceutical Care and Safe and Effective Medication Use." In MacKinnon N.J., ed., *Safe and Effective: The Eight Essential Elements of an Optimal Medication-Use System*. Ottawa, ON: Canadian Pharmacists Association.

48 Chang F. 2007.

49 The Pharmacy Group. 2008.

50 Ibid.

51 Management Committee. 2008. *Moving Forward: Pharmacy Human Resources for the Future*. Pharmacy Human Resources Challenges and Priorities: Perspectives of Pharmacy Students. Ottawa, ON: Canadian Pharmacists Association.

52 Ibid.

53 Romanow, R. May 12, 2002. Speaking about the Commission on the Future of Health Care in Canada at the Canadian Pharmacists Association Conference, Winnipeg, MB.

54 Canadian Medical Association and the Canadian Pharmaceutical Association. 1996. Joint Statement on Approaches to Enhancing the Quality of Drug Therapy. Ottawa, ON.

55 American College of Physicians–American Society of Internal Medicine. 2002. "Pharmacist Scope of Practice." *Annals of Internal Medicine* 136:79–85.

56 Canadian Institute for Health Information. 2009. *Drug Expenditure in Canada, 1985 to 2008*. Ottawa, ON: CIHI.

57 Wu J.Y.F., Leung W.Y.S., Chang S., Lee B., Zee B., Tong P.C.Y. et al. 2006. "Effectiveness of Telephone Counselling by a Pharmacist in Reducing Mortality in Patients Receiving Polypharmacy: Randomised Controlled Trial." *British Medical Journal* 333(7567):522.

58 Rickles N.M., Svarstad B.L., Statz-Paynter J.L., Taylor L.V., Kobak K.A. 2005. "Pharmacist Telemonitoring of Antidepressant Use: Effects on Pharmacist-Patient Collaboration. *Journal of the American Pharmacists Association* 45(3): 344–353.

59 Bunting B.A., Cranor C.W. 2006. "The Asheville Project: Long-Term Clinical, Humanistic, and Economic Outcomes of a Community-Based Medication Therapy Management Program for Asthma." *Journal of the American Pharmacists*

Association 46(2):133–147; Cranor C.W., Bunting B.A., Christensen D.B. 2003. "The Asheville Project: Long-Term Clinical and Economic Outcomes of a Community Pharmacy Diabetes Care Program." *Journal of the American Pharmaceutical Association* 43(2):173–184.

60 McLean W. 1998. "Pharmaceutical Care Evaluated: The Value of Your Services." *Canadian Pharmaceutical Journal* 131(4):34–40.

61 Dolovich L., Pottie K., Kaczorowski J., Farrell B., Austin Z., Rodriguez C. et al. 2008. "Integrating Family Medicine and Pharmacy to Advance Primary Care Therapeutics." *Clinical Pharmacology & Therapeutics* 83(6):913–917.

62 Ibid.

63 Pottie K., Farrell B., Haydt S., Dolovich L., Sellors C., Kennie N. et al. 2008. "Integrating Pharmacists into Family Practice Teams: Physicians' Perspectives on Collaborative Care." *Canadian Family Physician* 54(12):1714.

64 Tsuyuki R.T., Johnson J.A., Teo K.K., Simpson S.H., Ackman M.L., Biggs R.S. et al. 2002. "A Randomized Trial of the Effect of Community Pharmacist Intervention on Cholesterol Risk Management: The Study of Cardiovascular Risk Intervention by Pharmacists (SCRIP)." *Archives of Internal Medicine* 162(10):1149–1155.

65 Sinclair H.K., Bond C.M., Stead L.F. 2004. "Community Pharmacy Personnel Interventions for Smoking Cessation." *Cochrane Database of Systematic Reviews* (online) 1(1):CD003698.

66 Blenkinsopp A., Anderson C., Armstrong M. 2003. "Systematic Review of the Effectiveness of Community Pharmacy-Based Interventions to Reduce Risk Behaviours and Risk Factors for Coronary Heart Disease." *Journal of Public Health* 25(2):144–153.

67 Guidelines for pharmacy-based immunization advocacy [American Pharmacists Association website]. Available at http://www.pharmacist.com/am/Template.cfm?Section=Pharmacist_Immuniza tion_Center1&Template=/TaggedPage/TaggedPageDisplay.cfm&TPLID=126&Co ntentID=20733

68 Gatewood S., Goode J.V.R., Stanley D. 2006. "Keeping Up-to-Date on Immunizations: A Framework and Review for Pharmacists." *Journal of the American Pharmacists Association* 46(2):183–192.

69 Bowles S.K., Strang R.A., Wissemann E., Black E.K. 2006. "Evaluation of a Pilot Program of Community Pharmacy-Based Influenza Immunization Clinics." *Canadian Journal of Infectious Diseases and Medical Microbiology* 17:362.

70 Steyer T.E., Ragucci K.R., Pearson W.S., Mainous A.G. 2004. "The Role of Pharmacists in the Delivery of Influenza Vaccinations." *Vaccine* 22(8):1001–1006.

71 Botelho R.J., Dudrak R. 1992. "Home Assessment of Adherence to Long-Term Medication in the Elderly." *Journal of Family Practice* 35(1):61–65; Van Eijken M., Tsang S., Wensing M., de Smet P.A.G.M., Grol R.P.T.M. 2003. "Interventions to Improve Medication Compliance in Older Patients Living in the Community: A Systematic Review of the Literature." *Drugs & Aging* 20(3):229.

72 DiMatteo M.R., Giordani P.J., Lepper H.S., Croghan T.W. 2002. "Patient Adherence and Medical Treatment Outcomes: A Meta-analysis." *Medical Care* 40: 794–811.

73 Haynes R., Yao X., Degani A., Kripalani S., Garg A., McDonald H. 2005. "Interventions for Enhancing Medication Adherence" (review). *Cochrane Database of Systematic Reviews, Issue 4.*

74 MedsCheck. 2009. Available at http://www.health.gov.on.ca/cs/medscheck/index.html

75 Medication Review Service. 2008. Available at http://www.gov.ns.ca/health/Pharmacare/info_pro/pharmacists_bulletins/pharma_bulletins/Pharmacists%20Bulletin%202008-04.pdf.

76 De Smet P.A.G.M., Dautzenberg M. 2004. "Repeat Prescribing: Scale, Problems and Quality Management in Ambulatory Care Patients." *Drugs* 64(16):1779.

77 Lowe C.J., Raynor D.K., Purvis J., Farrin A., Hudson J. 2000. "Effects of a Medicine Review and Education Programme for Older People in General

Practice." *British Journal of Clinical Pharmacology* 50(2):172.

78 Kondro W. 2007. "Canada's Doctors Assail Pharmacist Prescribing." *Canadian Medical Association Journal* 177(6):558.

79 Canadian Medical Association. 2007. *Pharmacist Prescribing.* e-Panel Survey Summary. Available at www.cma.ca/index.cfm/ci_id/88902/la_id/1.htm.

80 Aharony L., Strasser S. 1993. "Patient Satisfaction: What We Know About and What We Still Need to Explore." *Medical Care Review* 50(1):49–79.

81 Larson L.N. 1998. "Patient Satisfaction with Delivery of Products and Information by an Ambulatory Care Pharmacy." *American Journal of Health-System Pharmacy* 55:1025–29; Kradjan W.A., Schulz R., Christensen D.B. et al. 1999. "Patients' Perceived Benefit from and Satisfaction with Asthma Related Pharmacy Services." *Journal of the American Pharmacists Association* 39:658–66; Johnson J.A., Coons S.L., Hays R.D. 1989. "The Structure of Satisfaction with Pharmacy Services. *Medical Care* 27:522–36; Cheng C.M. 2004. "Simple Additions to the Pharmacy Waiting Area May Increase Patient Satisfaction." *Journal of the American Pharmacists Association* 44:630–32; Amsler M.R., Murray M.D., Tierney W.M. et al. 2001. "Pharmaceutical Care in Chain Pharmacies: Beliefs and Attitudes of Pharmacists and Patients." *Journal of the American Pharmacists Association* 41:850–55; Larson L.N., Rovers J.P., MacKeigan L.D. 2002. "Patient Satisfaction with Pharmaceutical Care: Update of a Validated Instrument." *Journal of the American Pharmacists Association* 42:44–50; Nau D.P., Ried L.D., Lipowski E.E. et al. 2000. "Patients' Perceptions of the Benefits of Pharmaceutical Care." *Journal of the American Pharmacists Association* 40:36–40; Ried L.D., Wang F., Young H. et al. 1999. "Patients' Satisfaction and Their Perception of the Pharmacist." *Journal of the American Pharmacists Association* 39:835–42; Huyghebaert T., Farris K.B., Volume C.I. 1999. "Insights from Alberta Community Pharmacists." *Canadian Pharmacists Journal* 132(1):41–44.

82 Ried L.D. et al. 1999.

Chapter 7

83 Canadian Institute for Health Information. 2005. *Understanding Emergency Department Wait Times: Who Is Using Emergency Departments and How Long Are*

They Waiting? Ottawa, ON: CIHI.

84 Schoen C., Osborn, R., Huynh P., Doty M., Davis K., Zapert K., Peugh K., 2004. "Primary Care and Health System Performance: Adults. Experiences in Five Countries." *Health Affairs* (Web Exclusive) W4-487–503.

85 Canadian Institute for Health Information. 2005.

86 Zed P., Abu-Laban R., Balen R., Loewen P., Hohl C., Brubacher J., Wilbur K., Wiens M., Samoy L., Lacaria K., Purssel R., 2008. "Incidence, Severity and Preventability of Medication-Related Visits to the Emergency Department: A Prospective Study." *Canadian Medical Association Journal* 178:1563–69.

87 Ackroyd-Stolarz S., Guernsey J., MacKinnon N., Kovacs G. 2008. "Is a Prolonged Stay in the Emergency Department Associated with Adverse Events in Older Patients?" *Canadian Journal of Emergency Medicine* 10(3):259–60.

88 National Physician Survey. 2007. Available at www.nationalphysiciansurvey.ca.

89 Schoen C., Osborn R., Doty M.M., Bishop M., Peugh J., Murukutla N. 2007. "Toward Higher-Performance Health Systems: Adults' Health Care Experiences in Seven Countries." *Health Affairs* 26(6):w717–34.

90 National Physician Survey. 2007.

91 2005 National Survey of the Work and Health of Nurses, Statistics Canada and Canadian Institute for Heath Information. Shields, M., and Wilkins, K., 2009. "Factors Related to On-the-Job Abuse of Nurses by Patients." Statistics Canada.

92 Crilly J, Chobayer W, Creedy D. 2004, "Violence Toward Emergency Department Nurses by Patients." Accident and Emergency Nursing 12(2): 67–73

93 Canadian Institute for Health Information. 2005.

94 Alter D., Basinski A., and Naylor D., 1998. "A Survey of Provider Experiences and Perceptions of Preferential Access to Cardiovascular Care in Ontario, Canada." *Annals of Internal Medicine* 129:567–72.

95 Friedman S., Schofield L., and Tirkos S. et al. 2007. "Do As I Say, Not As I Do: A Survey of Public Impressions of Queue-Jumping and Preferential Access." *European Journal of Emergency Medicine* 14:260–264.

Chapter 8

96 Statistics Canada. "Number of Public Hospitals and Benevolent Institutions in Canada, Selected Years from 1923 to 1927." In Statistics Canada, *The Canada Yearbook 1927/1928*. Available at www65.statcan.gc.ca/acybo2/1927/acybo2_19270955001a-eng.htm.

97 Shouldice Hospital. www.shouldice.com.

98 Canadian Institute for Health Information. 2009. *National Health Expenditure Trends, 1975 TO 2009*. Ottawa, ON: CIHI.

99 Canadian Press. August 21, 2000. "Rundown hospital endangers patients." *The Daily News*. J. September 25, 2000. "Health Spending Increased." *Maclean's*.

100 Hardt K. April 9, 2009. "$15.3-Million Renovation for Kootenay Lake Hospital." Interior Health media release.

101 Hardt K. December 14, 2009. "KLH Redevelopment Construction Begins." Interior Health media release.

102 Canadian Institute for Health Information. 2007. *HSMR: A New Approach for Measuring Hospital Mortality Trends in Canada*. Ottawa, ON: CIHI.

103 MacKinnon N.J., Hartnell N.R., Metge C.J., Sketris I., Bussières J.F. 2008. "Medication Management: Perceptions and Opinions of Canadian Hospital Executives." *Canadian Journal of Hospital Pharmacy*. 61(1):41–48.

104 Huth E.J., Murray T.J. 2000. *Medicine in Quotations. Views of Health and Disease Through the Ages*. Philadelphia, PA: American College of Physicians.

105 Ibid.

106 Maxwell J. 2000. *Developing the Leader Within You*, 2nd ed. Nashville, TN: Thomas Nelson Publishers.

107 Baker G.R., Norton P.G., Flintoft V. et al. 2004. "The Canadian Adverse Events Study: The Incidence of Adverse Events Among Hospital Patients in Canada." *Canadian Medical Association Journal* 170:1678–86.

108 Ackroyd-Stolarz S., Read Guernsey J., MacKinnon N.J., Kovacs G. 2009. "Adverse Events in Older Patients Admitted to Acute Care: A Preliminary Cost Description." *Healthcare Management FORUM* 22(4): 32–36.

109 Center for Medicare and Medicaid Services. July 31, 2008. "Medicare and Medicaid Move Aggressively to Encourage Greater Patient Safety in Hospitals and Reduce Never Events." Press release. www.cmh.hhs.gov.

110 Zed P.J., Abu-Laban R.B., Balen R.M. et al. 2008. "Incidence, Severity and Preventability of Medication-Related Visits to the Emergency Department: A Prospective Study." *Canadian Medical Association Journal* 178:1563–69.

111 MacKinnon N.J et al. 2008.

112 Kopp B.J., Erstad B.L., Allen M.E. et al. 2006. "Medication Errors and Adverse Drug Events in an Intensive Care Unit: Direct Observation Approach for Detection." *Critical Care Medicine* 34(2):415–25.

113 Turple J., MacKinnon N.J., Davis B. 2006. "Frequency and Type of Medication Discrepancies in One Tertiary Care Hospital." *Healthcare Quarterly* 9:119–123.

114 Chevalier B.A.M., Parker D.S., MacKinnon N.J., Sketris I. 2006. "Nurses' Perceptions of Medication Safety and Medication Reconciliation Practices." *Canadian Journal of Nursing Leadership* 19(3):57–68.

115 Kaboli P.J., Hoth A., McClimon B.J., Schnipper J.L. 2006. "Clinical Pharmacists and Inpatient Medical Care: A Systematic Review." *Archives of Internal Medicine* 166(9):955–964; Kwan Y., Fernandes O.A., Nagge J.J., Wong G.G., Huh J.H., Hurn D.A. et al. 2007. "Pharmacist Medication Assessments in a Surgical Preadmission Clinic." *Archives of Internal Medicine* 167(10):1034–1040; Nickerson A., MacKinnon N.J., Roberts N., Saulnier L. 2005. "Drug-Therapy Problems, Inconsistencies and Omissions Identified During a Medication Reconciliation and Seamless Care Service." *Healthcare Quarterly* 8:65–72.

116 Leape L.L., Cullen D.J., Dempsey Clapp M. et al. 1999. "Pharmacist Participation on Physician Rounds and Adverse Drug Events in the Intensive Care Unit." *Journal of the American Medical Association* 281:267–70.

117 Bond C.A., Raehl C.L. 2007. "Clinical Pharmacy Services, Pharmacy Staffing, and Hospital Mortality Rates." *Pharmacotherapy* 27(4):481–493.

118 Kaboli P.J. et al. 2006.

119 Perez A., Doloresco F., Hoffman J.M., Meek P.D., Touchette D.R., Vermeulen L.C., Schumock G.T. 2008. "Economic Evaluations of Clinical Pharmacy Services: 2001–2005." *Pharmacotherapy* 28(11):285e–323e.

120 Avorn J. 1997. "Putting Adverse Drug Events into Perspective." *Journal of the American Medical Association* 277(4):341–342.

121 Hartnell N.R., MacKinnon N.J., Jones E.J.M., Genge R., Nestel M.D.M. 2006. "Perceptions of Patients and Health Care Professionals about Factors Contributing to Medication Errors and Potential Areas for Improvement." *Canadian Journal of Hospital Pharmacy* 59:177–83.

122 Ibid.

123 *Ghost Town.* 2008. Dreamworks SKG.

124 Chafe R., Levinson W., Sullivan T. 2009. "Disclosing Errors that Affect Multiple Patients." *Canadian Medical Association Journal* 180(11):1125–27.

125 Jauhar S. January 1, 2008. "Explain a Medical Error? Sure. Apologize Too?" *The New York Times.*

Chapter 9

126 Morrissey S.P., Whyte A. 2009. "Something Is Squeezing My Skull." *Years of Refusal.* Decca Records.

127 Content based on a modified version of a table found in: Wallston K. 2007. "Patient Participation and Intelligent Adherence." In MacKinnon N.J., ed., *Safe*

and Effective: The Eight Essential Elements of an Optimal Medication-Use System. Ottawa, ON: Canadian Pharmacists Association.

128 Moerman D.E. 2002. *Meaning, Medicine and the 'Placebo Effect.'* Cambridge, UK: Cambridge University Press.

129 Ibid.

130 Gould O.N., Todd L., Irvine-Meek J. 2009. "Adherence Devices in a Community Sample: How Are Pillboxes Used?" *Canadian Pharmacists Journal* 142:28–35.

131 Flanagan P.S., MacKinnon N.J., Hanlon N., Robertson H. 2002. "Identification of Intervention Strategies to Reduce Preventable Drug-Related Morbidity in Older Adults." *Geriatrics Today: Journal of the Canadian Geriatrics Society* 5(2):76–80.

132 Hepler C.D., Grainger-Rousseau T. 1995. "Pharmaceutical Care versus Traditional Drug Treatment." *Drugs* 49:1–10.

133 MacKinnon N.J., Hartnell N.R., Bowles S.K., Kirkland S.A., Jones E.J.M. 2006. "Incident-Event Rate of Preventable Drug-Related Morbidity in Older Adults in Nova Scotia." *Canadian Journal of Geriatrics* 9(5):159–163.

134 Holbrook A., Thabane L., Keshavjee K., Dolovich L., Bernstein B. et al. 2009. "Individualized Electronic Decision Support and Reminders to Improve Diabetes Care in the Community: COMPETE II Randomized Trial." *Canadian Medical Association Journal* 181(1–2): 37–44.

Chapter 10

135 "Climategate: What the Climate Scientists Wrote and When They Wrote It." November 24, 2009. *Financial Post.*

136 Associated Press. December 3, 2004. "Police Recover Doughnuts." *USA Today*; Nguyen T. December 3, 2004. "Police follow doughnuts to stolen truck." www.fleetowner.com.

137 Winterstein A.G., Kimberlin C.L. November 4, 2008. "Expert and Consumer Evaluation of Consumer Medication Information — 2008." Final Report to the U.S. Department of Health and Human Services and the Food and Drug Administration.

Chapter 11

138 Canadian Cancer Society. 2009. *Cancer Drug Access for Canadians.* Available at http://www.cancer.ca/Canada-wide/About%20us/Media%20centre/CW-Media%20releases/CW-2009/~/media/CCS/Canada%20wide/Files%20List/Engli sh%20files%20heading/pdf%20not%20in%20publications%20section/CAN-CER%20DRUG%20ACCESS%20FINAL%20-%20English.ashx

139 Health Council of Canada. 2009. *The National Pharmaceuticals Strategy: A Prescription Unfilled.* Status Report and Commentary. Toronto, ON: Health Council.

140 Waterman A.D., Gallagher T.H., Garbutt J. et al. 2006. "Brief Report: Hospitalized Patients' Attitudes About and Participation in Error Prevention." *Journal of General Internal Medicine.* April 2006; 21(4):367–370.

141 Montague T. 2004. *Patients First: Closing the Health Care Gap in Canada.* Toronto, ON: John Wiley & Sons Canada Ltd.

142 Wikipedia. http://en.wikipedia.org/wiki/Ignaz_Semmelweis.

143 Matherne B. *A Reader's Journal.* Available at www.doyletics.com/arj/tcat-crvw.htm.

144 Thompson M. 1949. *The Cry and the Covenant.* New York City, NY: Garden City Books.

145 Australian Institute of Policy & Science. Available at www.aips.net.au/97.html.

146 The Nobel Prize in Physiology or Medicine 2005. Press release. Available at http://nobelprize.org/nobel_prizes/medicine/laureates/2005/press.html.

147 Wright O. January 2, 2004. "15 Cardiologists on Airplane as Woman Has Heart Attack." *Halifax Chronicle-Herald*; "Heart attack woman on plane — 15 cardiologists on board." January 2, 2004. *Medical News Today* (online). Available at www.medicalnewstoday.com/articles/5118.php.

INDEX

ACKNOWLEDGEMENTS

We are grateful to the following individuals for their invaluable contributions.

Stacy Ackroyd-Stolarz, Susan Biali, Susan Borgersen, Jane Buss, Chris Church, Louise Cloutier, Marc Cote, Erin Creasey, Jack David, Alison DeLory, Mark Embrett, Cindy Forbes, Elizabeth Foy, Christopher Goguen, Anne Greer, Sean Higgins, Tannis Jurgens, Jocelyn LeClerc, Daphna Levit, Paula Levy, Mary MacCara, Helena MacLean, Karen MacPherson, Ron MacPherson, Steve Morgan, Tiffany Nguyen, Joshua O'Hagan, Grant Perry, John Pugsley, Guylaine Roy, Syr Ruus, Andrea Scobie, Kim Sears, Ann Thompson, Gordon Wright.

OK, I confess. I had help. Buckets of it.

A decade ago, on a whim, I signed up for a creative writing course and I would like to extend my deepest gratitude to my teachers and mentors Beth Munroe, Peggie Graham, Carol Bruneau, and Gwen Davies for their sage advice and encouragement early in my writing career. I would also like to thank the editorial staff at the *Medical Post*, particularly Colin Leslie, Joe McAllister, and Rick Campbell for their support of my writing and of physician writers in general. The wonderful and witty Jane Buss, former executive director of the Writers Federation of Nova Scotia, stepped up to the plate when we were in need of a little writerly advice. Kudos to Neil MacKinnon, my partner in this venture, for the kernel of an idea that grew into this book. My Wednesday writing group Helena MacLean, Susan Borgersen, Anne Greer, Syr Ruus, Daphna Levit, and Gordon Wright read endless drafts and told me what should hit the printed page what should hit the recycle bin. You guys rock! The old adage that if you need something done you should ask a busy person certainly held true as physician colleagues Louise Cloutier, Cindy Forbes, and Susan Biali provided timely and invaluable content feedback content on several chapters. Thank you to Jack David at ECW for his belief in our project, and to the patient and talented staff at ECW, particularly Erin Creasey, who moved this project from our keyboards to the book you are now holding. My wonderful patients have granted me the privilege of helping them navigate their own personal health needs, and I am grateful for the opportunity to continue to learn from them every day.

On a personal note, I am so very lucky to have the world's best parents, Karen and Ron MacPherson, who served as early readers and cheerleaders — and so much more. And of course, I owe a huge debt of gratitude to my husband, Chris, and our children, Ben and Sophie, for their endless love and support.

Finally, there is one individual for whom words will never be enough. A huge shout out goes to our editor, the incomparable Alison DeLory. Heartfelt thanks, Alison, for your dedication, energy and enthusiasm, as well as for all the times you talked me down off a ledge during the writing of this book.

Rhonda Church, M.D.

The latin Clan MacKinnon motto, *audentes fortuna juvat*, can be translated into English as "fortune (good luck) aids the daring or brave." In many ways, this may well sum up our experience in writing *Take as Directed*. With some notable exceptions, authors are not typically characterized as being daring or brave. However, taking on something as complex and overwhelming as the Canadian healthcare system may indeed garner someone the title of being daring or brave. Or, as some might suggest, foolish.

Joking aside, our goal in creating *Take as Directed* was to drawn upon our experience as health professionals and, in my case, a health-care educator and researcher, to convey tips and advice in a practical, user-friendly way. You can be the judge as to whether we have succeeded at our attempt to do this. While I write on a daily basis in my role as a Professor at Dalhousie University and I have previously edited two books for health professionals, *Take as Directed* proved to be a formidable challenge. In this case, our good fortune was to be blessed with the input from many individuals who are acknowledged by name.

As Rhonda has done above, I would like to single out the critical role of Alison DeLory who worked with me from the early days of *Take as Directed* when it was a very rough idea, providing valuable guidance right through the entire process. Alison also suggested a potential co-author for the book; a family physician who was a talented writer from — who would believe it — my hometown of Bridgewater, Nova Scotia. Rhonda proved to be that and much more; an engaging and caring person who ended up being the engine driving the writing process. She carried on her writing at an even pace even through the challenges of maintaining her family practice and dealing with the H1N1 crisis.

Rhonda and I also had the good fortune to find an excellent partner in ECW Press. As Rhonda mentioned in her comments, Erin Creasey, in particular, has been supportive and enthusiastic throughout the entire process. I would like to thank ECW for taking a risk with us.

Finally, I would like to acknowledge the financial support we received in the form of an unrestricted educational grant to Dalhousie University from GlaxoSmithKline. Their support truly was unrestricted as they never asked to see a draft manuscript and simply believed in the idea and allowed Rhonda, Alison, and I to proceed with the writing.

Neil J. MacKinnon, Ph.D., FCSHP

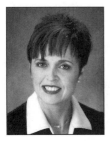

RHONDA L. CHURCH, M.D., has more than two decades of experience as a cradle-to-grave family physician. She is a Past President of Doctors Nova Scotia, the professional organization that represents the province's physicians and physicians-in-training to government, the public, and other health-care stakeholders. She is a past member of the Board of Directors of the Canadian Medical Association and currently chairs the Canadian Medical Association's Core Committee on Health Care and Promotion. Dr. Church resides in Bridgewater, N.S., with her husband and their two teenaged children.

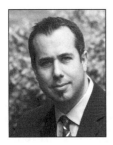

NEIL J. MACKINNON, PH.D., FCSHP, is Associate Director of Research, College of Pharmacy, and Professor, School of Health Administration and Department of Community Health and Epidemiology at Dalhousie University in Halifax. A Ph.D.-trained pharmacist, he has published more than 150 papers in pharmacy and medical literature and has given more than 140 presentations at health-care and scientific meetings on the safety and effectiveness of the medication-use system. He has been the lead investigator of several studies in this area, and he heads the largest research program in Canada that addresses the issue of medication errors. Neil is currently president of the Canadian Society of Hospital Pharmacists.